The Skin You Live In

The Skin You Live In

How to Recognize & Prevent Skin Problems
& Keep Your Skin Youthful & Attractive

NORMAN GOLDSTEIN, M.D.
F.A.C.P. DERMATOLOGY
in association with Robert B. Stone

Hart Publishing Company, Inc. • New York City

To Ruth, Heidi, and Rick

ISBN NO. 08055-1257-8 (PAPERBACK 08055-0341-2)
LIBRARY OF CONGRESS CATALOG CARD NO. 77-77093

MANUFACTURED IN THE UNITED STATES OF AMERICA

ACKNOWLEDGMENTS

I would like to express my sincere appreciation to Nancy Wilder, BPA, my photographic assistant; to Lynn Murakami, Vernon Koto, Al Saito, and Dede Chinn, my research assistants; to Doris Rosskopf, my secretary; to my office family: Aiko Yamamoto, Arleen Snyder, Alva Takahashi, Aileen Isono, Doris Jones, and Doreen Takemoto; to the Dermatologists of Hawaii; to the Hawaii Medical Library; to the American Cancer Society; to the Honolulu Medical Group Research and Education Foundation; to the Straub Clinic Research Foundation; to the many physicians who referred their patients to me, and most importantly to my patients and their skins.

Contents

List of Illustrations

How to Spot Serious Skin Trouble

Your skin is the house you live in. It keeps you warm or cool, protects you from the elements, and presents you to the world.

Like a house, your skin can be the envy of others—or an eyesore.

If your skin is your house, then in a sense, I as a dermatologist am your home-improvement specialist.

These days, doctors rarely make house calls. But consider this book as my visit to your house.

The primary purpose of my visit is to help you maintain an attractive, youthful, healthy skin.

Health and happiness go hand in hand. Skin health is where your trip begins. A lovely, healthy skin, for male or female alike, can be the key factor in love, business success, popularity, social acceptance, and self-image and emotional security.

Easy-to-make mistakes can cause serious skin problems. Popular misconceptions in the treatment of skin problems can leave lifetime scars.

Easy-to-learn skin care methods can halt unwanted skin conditions before they become serious problems, postpone telltale signs of aging, prevent blemishes, and keep you radiantly youthful and outstandingly attractive.

Prepare yourself for some surprises. You may be doing things to your skin that are aggravating the very condition that you wish to alleviate. Some so-called beauty aids may be beauty deterrents. Treatments that make you more youthful-looking today may be hastening your wrinkled tomorrow.

You need to know more about the skin you live in. As a practicing dermatologist, I am aghast, outraged, and saddened daily. Aghast at the misconceptions people have about the skin, outraged at some of the false claims made for certain skin products, and saddened by the sorrow and pain that are produced by ignorance about the skin.

My profession as a skin specialist is also a source of joy, pleasure, and gratification. Joy when a formerly acne-ridden teenager returns for a checkup with clean, attractive facial skin—and a big smile. Pleasure when a middle-aged woman returns looking in her twenties. Gratification when a skin cancer is spotted and removed, and serious trouble is thus prevented.

A beautiful and vibrant skin is important; it is the focus of every chapter that lies ahead. But it is the prevention of serious skin problems to which we must give first priority.

This chapter will alert you to the danger signs of skin trouble. The chapters that follow tackle the most serious of these problems—for example, acne, psoriasis, and skin cancer. Then, we get into minor skin problems, such as allergies and blemishes. Finally, we get into the preventive and positive steps that you can take to make a good skin even better.

How to Be a Skin Vigilante

We all look in the mirror. Men and women alike look in the mirror more than once a day. But I have news for you, and I am going to let you find it out for yourself. Read the next sentence, then close your eyes.

With your eyes closed, picture first a banana; then erase the banana and picture a close friend; finally, picture your own face. (Put the book down, close your eyes, and do it now.)

Thank you. I am quite sure you had no trouble picturing the banana. Even your friend's face probably showed up very recognizably. But I'll wager that your own face was not that easy to "see."

When we look at ourselves in the mirror, we usually take our reflections for granted. We check the hair, the complexion, the makeup, the necktie, etc. We really know less about our own faces than we do about our neighbors' faces.

I ask that you get to know your own face better. I ask that when you look in the mirror, you take a closer look. I ask that you go over your facial skin as you might go over a street map.

I ask that you become a skin vigilante.

Of course, it is not just the skin on your face that you will be watching, but the face is our most vulnerable area socially. Your complexion deserves more of your vigilance than other areas of your skin. But your whole skin—back, legs, arms, chest, neck—all will come under your scrutiny.

The purpose of your vigilance is to spot small changes now, so as to avoid big problems later. Avoiding big problems later can pay off in hard cash, love, the addition of youthful years, and a happier life.

This preventative skin care can be accomplished by you at home in most cases. In some cases skin care will require help from your physician or dermatologist.

Do not be embarrassed to see your dermatologist on what might turn out to be a minor matter. He will be glad to instruct you in self-care. Of course, if your skin problem turns out to require more skilled assistance, like strong medication or even minor surgery, your doctor will want to treat the condition before it gets out of control and requires more intensive procedures; and before the condition causes you discomfort, disability, or disfigurement.

Let's make a quick survey of what you should be checking out as a skin vigilante.

Some Major Skin Problems

You are looking at your face in the mirror. You see a blackhead. You use a cleansing cream. Right? Wrong! You are adding to the causative factor that brought about the first blackhead—oil.

Somewhere at this very minute, somebody is treating blackheads with oil-based preparations and encouraging acne. Somebody is putting coconut oil on the skin for sun protection and getting no protection at all. Somebody is watching a mole turn black and passing it off as nothing, when actually the mole may signal cancer. Somebody is using twice the prescribed amount of medication on psoriasis to speed results, when actually such over-medication can make psoriasis worse.

Somewhere, somebody is using a spray on contact dermatitis symptoms. The most common of these symptoms in the United States are poison ivy, oak, and sumac. In Hawaii, the most common symptom is mango. Some sprays will cause contact dermatitis to get worse.

Hopefully, you will read this book all the way through rather than just those chapters that seem pertinent to your skin now. Educate yourself about the skin you live in. Learn what problems exist, and the correct way to treat them should you ever be faced with such problems in the future.

Let's examine acne. Not a pretty condition to examine. But we begin with acne because it is the most common skin condition that dermatologists are called upon to treat.

If you become a skin vigilante, chances are you can prevent acne from getting as great a foothold on your skin as it gets in the majority of cases that wind up in dermatologists' offices.

There are a number of over-the-counter preparations that are sold to acne sufferers that do not help acne; in fact, some medications can make acne worse. Also, there are a number of non-prescription preparations at your local pharmacy that are helpful to acne.

Did you know that most acne starts with blackheads? And did you know that there is an inexpensive tool that you can get at your pharmacy to remove blackheads?

We are going to devote the next chapter to acne—what to look for, and what to do when you find it. Also, how to minimize the progressive effects of acne.

Acne can be a disaster for otherwise attractive individuals. Another skin condition can be so sad it is called a heartbreak—the heartbreak of psoriasis.

Psoriasis need not be a tragedy; but it is a serious enough condition to merit a whole chapter in this book. The chapter on psoriasis will hopefully take the heartbreak out of this skin problem for psoriatic readers.

Another chapter covers the sun as a cause of skin cancer. The thrust of this discussion on the sun is how to prevent the cumulative effect of sunlight from causing skin cancer. However, you may unknowingly be putting some chemical on your skin (or taking some drug internally) that will make your skin so sensitive to the sun that one mild exposure can be harmful.

A skier in Colorado notices brown or tan patches on her skin. A sun-worshiper, she had never noticed any harmful effects before. But—she has just gone on an oral contraceptive.

A Minneapolis senior citizen has been troubled with anxiety. He takes a walk in the mild winter sun. That evening, he notices an eruption on his face. He does not connect it with the tranquilizer he has been taking.

A mother takes her newborn infant outdoors for some fresh air and sunlight. Within a few hours the baby's skin has broken out with red inflamed splotches.

The oral contraceptive is a photosensitizer. The old gentleman's tranquilizer contained phenothiazine—a photosensitizer. The infant's hospital soap contained hexachlorophene—another photosensitizer.

Are these the only three photosensitizers that we should know about? No, there are hundreds.

One photosensitizer, the cyclamates, used in low calorie drinks, is no longer a hazard, because it has been banned. An after shave lotion—like Jade East—could also be a sun-sensitizer. A perfume—like Shalimar—could be a sun-sensitizer.

Other photosensitizers are still around in some antibacterial soaps, deodorant soaps, tranquilizers, and antibiotics. There are photosensitizing chemicals in some hair dyes and bleaches, antihistamines, insecticides, oil-based cosmetics, and products containing tar derivatives.

Skin that is supersensitive to the sun may also be the result of an internal disorder, metabolic or otherwise. If no chemical is obviously the culprit, see your doctor.

Skin that has become supersensitive to even mild sunlight is skin that will be aged by the sun super fast. On your guard, vigilante!

Your Dermatologist as an Experienced Vigilante

If you are in doubt about the nature of what you are seeing or feeling on your skin, and if the condition persists, it is wise to see your physician or dermatologist.

The rash you see or the itch you feel may be a skin (and only skin) problem, such as those that we are discussing in these pages. But the skin you live in frequently reflects what is going on inside other parts of your body (and mind, as we will later discuss).

A dermatologist can frequently see subtle evidence on the skin of such not-so-subtle conditions as leukemia, diabetes, anemia, or venereal disease. By your skin's color, he might detect kidney or liver problems, or vitamin deficiencies due either to diet or metabolic imbalance.

A dermatologist can see in the folds of the skin or on the cuticles of the nails, or on the surface of the tongue, or on the eyeball signs of internal problems. Problems quickly treated are problems more quickly and easily removed.

When an internal problem is suspected by your dermatologist on preliminary examination, he may do a biopsy or a blood test for laboratory confirmation, and then refer you to an internist or surgeon for further evaluation.

All of this is beyond the scope of this book, but at this point a word to the wise vigilante is in order: Make an occasional checkup by your physician or dermatologist part of your program for healthy skin.

More than likely a rash, boil, itch, or blister will prompt that visit.

We see a lot of fever blisters. The technical term is herpes simplex. Herpes simplex is caused by a virus that makes its home on the skin or in the nerve below the skin. There the virus stays for prolonged periods of time, many months—and for some people, years.

When your body resistance is weakened by stress, sun exposure, common cold, or other illness, the virus's effects on your skin become pronounced. The presence of the virus becomes observable and felt—as a cold sore or fever blister.

Usually, cold sores occur on the lower lip, when sun strikes the hardest. Fever blisters can appear on a finger. In these locations, herpes simplex generally causes no problems. Cold packs are the simplest and most effective treatment for these manifestations of herpes simplex.

Occasionally, a man gets a fever blister on his penis—an emotional and sexual disaster. The disaster is usually compounded by the fact that these men are vulnerable to stress—which is probably a causative factor in the first place. But the additional sexual crisis caused by the eruption of herpes simplex on these high-strung, complusive people makes the fever blister in this location an emotional trauma.

Herpes simplex usually disappears in five to ten days, even without treatment. An over-the-counter treatment is Blistex—a jelly in lipstick form. Antibiotics and cortisone injections are more potent methods of attack.

A recent technique to combat herpes simplex is called photoinactivation. You apply a dye to the skin and then expose it to light, such as an incandescent bulb. The dye is sensitive to the light, and inactivates the herpes simplex virus in a few days.

Notice that I said "inactivates." None of these methods does more than that. The herpes simplex virus survives, to strike again when your resistance is lowered.

Photoinactivation is under suspicion for being cancer-inducing, and many dermatologists are not using it for that reason. Ether or chloroform, both lipid solvents, also inactivate the virus. They do this by dissolving the capsule with which the virus surrounds itself. The blister then dries up. Again, there is no real cure for the virus; it just becomes temporarily inactive.

When you get right down to it, those cold packs are a good bet. Apply an ice cube to the cold sore or blister. The virus goes into "hibernation." If the lesions left by the blister are a problem, your dermatologist can freeze them with ethyl chloride or liquid nitrogen.

Simple rule: If you have a fever blister, treat it with ice. If it persists more than five to seven days, see your physician or dermatologist. If the blister returns more frequently than once or twice a year, or if it appears in especially sensitive areas like the eye—where it can cause blindness—or the sexual organs—where, in women, it has increased the incidence of cervical cancer—see your family physician or a dermatologist.

Also, what looks like simple fever blister can be something more serious—cancer. One soldier, age forty, had a blister on his lower lip, and because it kept returning but then healing, he assumed it was herpes simplex. Possibly it was, at the beginning. But besides being out in the sun a lot, this man was a pipe smoker. The stem of a pipe, through constant friction and heat, often induces lip cancer. Combined with herpes simplex, exposure to sunlight and pipe smoking had contributed in this case to cause cancer and necessitate an operation.

Certain activities and occupations are, as the surgeon general proclaims on hundreds of millions of cigarette packages, dangerous to your health. Cigarette smoke can cause lung cancer. Pipe smoking can cause lip cancer.

Years ago, chimney sweeping was a hazardous occupation for men. The smoke residues got onto the clothing, then onto the skin of the scrotum, causing cancer of the scrotum.

Anybody today who works with carbon products, petroleum products, or arsenic products is exposing himself to the danger of skin cancer. In the southeastern United States, I once treated twin sons of a doctor, now both doctors themselves, for cancer on their hands and feet, because their father, some forty years before, meaning well, had given them tonics—pep medicines—containing arsenic.

Doctors and dentists who work with X-rays are risking skin cancer. Now you know why your dentist asks you to put your finger inside your mouth to hold the X-ray plate. Periodic X-rays are not harmful, but working with X-rays day in and day out is another matter.

Skin vigilantes need to be aware of "extra-ordinary" environmental conditions when they examine ordinary blemishes.

Shingles—Recognition and Treatment

Another virus—herpes zoster—causes shooting pains up and down the arm or leg or side of the face. Herpes zoster is called shingles, because it resembles a girdle or band around the body—usually half of the body.

The herpes zoster virus lives in the nerve, and wherever that nerve leads to becomes the pained and affected area.

The more severe the condition, the more the physician or dermatologist is alerted to a serious and more general malfunction that has lowered the body's resistance. Older people are frequently the victims of painful attacks of shingles, which may portend internal cancer.

Shingles can be pinhead blisters, sometimes growing to pea size. They can be filled with clear fluid or bloody fluid. The distribution of shingles follows the path of the nerve. Usually, shingles does not cross the mid-part of the body (as from left to right side) because of nerve geography.

An old wives' tale is that if shingles crosses from one side of the body to the other, your days are numbered. It's the days of this tale that are numbered, because it is simply not true!

The only serious danger involved in shingles is if they lead to an infection because of scratching, etc., or if the patient is on chemotherapy for cancer, or on cortisone, as for arthritis: then the resistance is sharply lowered, and the shingles can become total over the entire body, and can be fatal.

As a skin vigilante, you can recognize shingles as tiny blisters. You might get these blisters on the ear lobe, or in front of the ear, or on the arms, legs, or thighs. Whenever you spot a patch of blisters, have your physician or dermatologist make a scraping and lab test. Changes in the blood cells are the tip-off.

Younger people get milder attacks of shingles than older people, and usually treatment takes care of the condition permanently. Shingles is more likely to be more widespread (and more painful) among older people. If shingles returns repeatedly in a younger adult, the chances are that resistance is being sapped by some other problem.

The treatment for shingles is a cortisone injection. The quicker you spot shingles, see your doctor, and have the injection, the less the post-herpes pain. This pain is the exorbitant price of shingles. The discomfort can be lasting and severe—a deep, gnawing nerve pain.

Everything we see in adults can take place in children, too. Children are not immune to shingles, psoriasis, or even venereal disease. All skin conditions can occur in all people.

Older people are more likely to get those skin conditions brought on by degeneration of the tissues or vital organs, but younger people, I'm sorry to say, are also vulnerable to such disorders.

Dark Spots, Light Spots—Pigmentation Problems

People of all races and skin colors can have problems with skin color. Skin pigmentation is affected by both external and internal factors. Sometimes the causes of pigmentation disorders are easily traced, sometimes not so easily.

It is just as alarming to a dark-skinned person when light spots appear, as it is to a light-skinned person when dark spots appear.

A young man of Japanese descent in Hawaii began to notice white patches on his back. The spots became quite large, and slightly raised. The youth was embarrassed to be seen on the beach. His dermatologist could not locate a simply physical cause, and concluded that the condition might be partly emotional in nature. The dermatologist suggested hypnotherapy. So the young man visited a physician who practiced hypnosis. The physician had the young man relax deeply. Then he gave the young man's subconscious mind "instructions" to restore his skin to its natural color. After one such session, the white areas became less raised and less noticeable. After three sessions, the young man was back on the beach.

Large areas of white spots constitute a condition called vitilito. Although often unrelated to internal problems, vitilito can be associated with anemia, diabetes, or thyroid imbalance. Check it out. It might be that the skin will not be treated, but rather the internal cause. If your doctor determines that your vitilito is solely a skin condition, he will probably use psoralen. Now synthesized, psoralen was originally an old Egyptian medicine made from grinding up the leaf of a certain plant, and was applied directly to the skin. Today, psoralen is a pill that you swallow.

White spots (Vitilito), before (left) *and after* (right) *treatment with psoralen.*

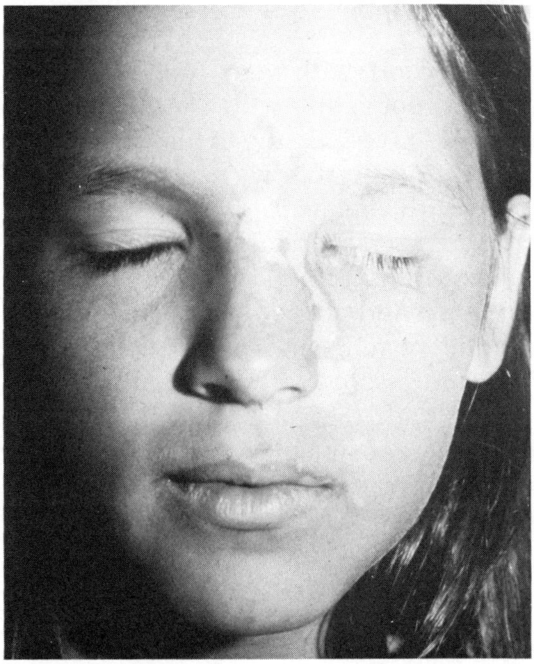

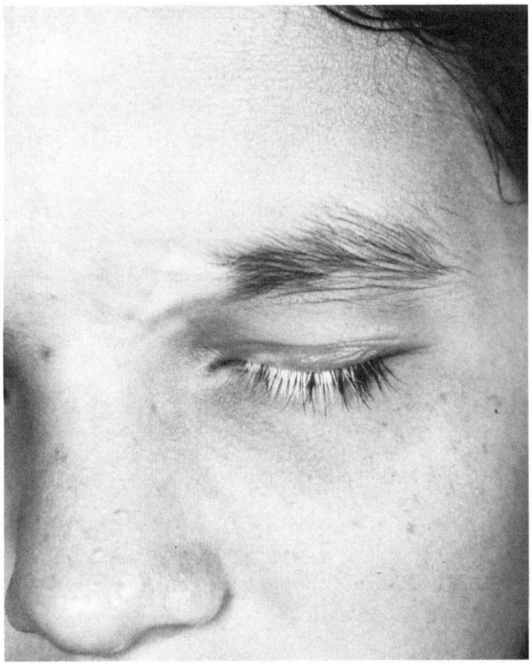

Vitilito is a total absence of color. It is not just a lighter patch, but a patch that is white and without any pigmentation. For instance, in Hawaii there is a fungus called kane; this fungus acts like a bandage on the skin and cuts out sunlight. Kane leaves a lighter patch, but the skin still has pigmentation, so it differs in looks from vitilito. We will discuss different fungus problems and how to treat them at home in a subsequent chapter.

Darker pigmentation is more common than lighter. A change of pigmentation around a mole, like a dark ring, is a danger sign. Spot it. Have it checked. More about moles later in this chapter, as they are important focal points for the skin vigilante.

Dark spots on the skin such as freckles, age spots, so-called liver spots, and even some mole-like areas are usually caused by the sun.

Freckles come and go with the sun. Liver spots and age spots have nothing to do with the liver, or your age. These blemishes show up after many years of skin exposure to the sun. An old person without such exposure is not likely to have these brown spots. Notice that the dark patches are usually on the backs of the hands, upper chest, forehead, face, and temples—where the sun hits most frequently.

Herrick called the sun "The glorious lamp of heaven." Freckled people might disagree. So might people with "liver" spots.

Some age spots can be scraped off with your finger. Try scraping the edge of an age or liver spot gently with your fingernail. You might find that the spot "gives" easily. If the spot is tenacious, do not attempt to remove it this way. Your dermatologist has safer treatments—with chemicals, bleaches, dermabrasion (a sandpapering-type process), or freezing.

Age spots can become pre-cancerous, and then cancerous. If age spots get thicker—and turn hard and crusted—they may no longer be innocent spots, and should be removed.

Cosmetically speaking, these dark spots are called age spots because they are closely affiliated with the years, and there is cosmetic advantage in removing them. Most bleaches sold over the counter are worthless. Eldoquin Forte is an over-the-counter bleaching cream that takes months to work, but it does lighten some freckles and age spots.

When you use any product like Eldoquin Forte that requires continuous application, you get faster results *not* by putting on more at a time; but by putting on less at a time, several more times a day.

Hormones stimulate pigmentation, and can produce dark spots on the skin. Hormones increase in the body at puberty and pregnancy—also, when the birth control pill is taken.

A pregnant woman frequently notices dark spots appearing at the nipples, cheeks, or center of the abdomen. The "mask of pregnancy" is the formation of these dark areas on the forehead, cheeks, and upper lip, often duplicated by birth control pills. These dark spots are nothing to be alarmed about.

If the dark areas remain for months after pregnancy and get progressively darker, they should be examined by your doctor.

These spots can be a "giveaway" that a woman is on birth control pills, so there may be a social or cosmetic reasons to see your doctor for treatment and removal.

Hormones can also accelerate hair growth. Excessive hair growth in an area can signal a hormone imbalance for male or female, and this imbalance is occasionally caused by a male hormone-producing tumor.

We will get into hair—both problems and beautification—in a later chapter.

What You Should Watch for in Moles

Beauty is only skin deep, they say. But that is deep enough for most people. I am covering problem areas of the skin first, because they are the greatest deterrents to beauty. Later, we will be more positive, and provide ways to make a healthy skin even more attractive.

If a dark spot appears on a woman's face, I call it a beauty mark. Anywhere else, it's a mole. Moles are ubiquitous, and by and large innocuous, but. . . .

Let's talk about the most dangerous moles first.

There is a mole that grows very fast. If you spot such a mole, you must move fast, too. This type of mole is insidious. It is called keratoacanthoma. Keratoacanthoma is a frightening kind of skin cancer, because it grows so fast.

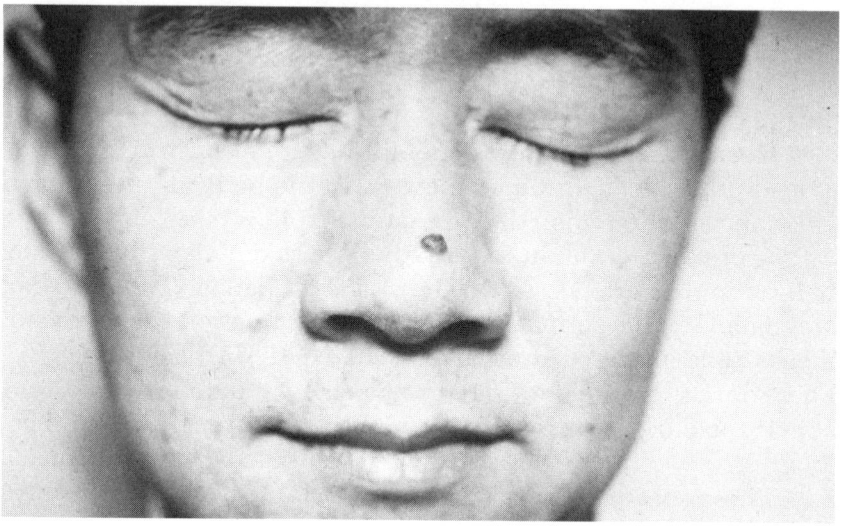

Benign mole on tip of nose.

In describing skin conditions, I will occasionally make a comparison with geographical conditions. There is a striking similarity in the kinds of changes that occur on the surface of the earth and on the surface of our bodies.

This fast-growing mole begins to look like a volcano. It has a crater in the center and a hard, horny crust around it, plus material in the center that appears to be about to erupt.

In a few weeks or months, this mole can grow to two or more inches in diameter. It grows down as well as on the surface, and that is what makes it so dangerous. The mole may heal itself. But then again, the mole may have grown so deep that it affects internal tissues. So do not depend on moles to be self-healing.

Dermatology journals have some classic cartoons exploiting the term "mole," and picturing it as an animal gnawing and burrowing on the skin. If any mole deserves this interpetation, it is this fast growing, deep-burrowing, potentially cancerous mole we call keratoacanthoma.

Most moles are present at birth, under the skin. As the person gets more sun exposure, the moles become larger, more elevated, and darker. Moles can exist in covered areas, but they are usually much darker in exposed areas—because of the sun.

The majority of moles do not ever need medical attention, do not need to be excised or cut out. If the mole is on your palm, sole of the foot, genitals, or some place where they is likely to be constant friction or irritation, there is a greater chance of it becoming cancerous. These are the moles that dermatologists will cut out most frequently, especially if there is a change in shape, size, or color.

Any mole that suddenly shows changes such as these is suspect. A mole might change its surface characteristics, for example, becoming crusty or starting to bleed. These could be signs of pre-cancerous or actually cancerous development.

A mole might grow hair. There is a common fallacy that hair on a mole should ring your alarm bell. Actually, a hairy mole does not have a good or a bad prognosis, except: a large mole that grows hair should be removed. By "large," I mean the so-called "bathing suit mole," which might be a few square inches or much larger in area. Bathing suit moles have a high incidence of skin cancer, and plastic surgeons usually cut them out at an early stage.

You, as a skin vigilante, should also observe irritation in the surrounding tissue of a mole. Sometimes these changes call your attention to them without your being that aware or vigilant—they begin to be painful. Such moles merit an appointment with your family physician or dermatologist.

Your doctor may merely put on a cortisone cream to quiet down the irritation for a week or two. That might take care of the irritation. If not, a biopsy is made to determine whether the mole is cancerous. If so, it may be frozen off.

An obsession with moles, however is a form of hypochondria. Most moles never become a problem. If dermatologists were asked to remove every mole, they would have time for nothing else. If surgeons were asked to remove every appendix, they would have time for nothing else. So, like the trouble-free appendix, the trouble-free mole lives out our lives with us.

When it is considered necessary to remove a suspicious mole, there are several ways it can be done. My own personal preference is to be conservative: to cut the mole level with the skin. This is often called a superficial removal. It is done with a local anesthetic like novocaine, and leaves a minimum of scar. A razor or scalpel is used, and the elevated part of the mole just slic-

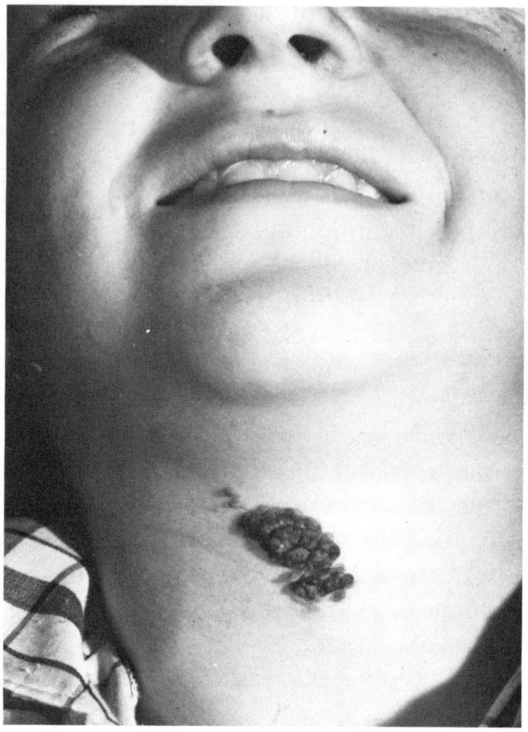

Warty mole on neck of twelve-year-old boy—bears watching.

ed away. A chemical is put on the skin to stop the bleeding, or an electric needle is used to seal the wound. The small, flat scar is usually skin-colored. Cryosurgery—freezing with liquid nitrogen—is another clean and quick method of mole removal.

The disadvantage of the freezing process is that it prevents the lab from making a biopsy. Most dermatologists seek a biopsy to check out the "nature" of the mole, or for that matter, of anything that is taken off the skin.

In certain places, like where there is a wrinkle or fold in the skin, the doctor may conduct a more thorough mole removal by excision. The mole will be excised—cut out—in an elliptical manner, and sutures will be used to bring the skin together, leaving a small scar.

Invariably, I am asked, "Doctor, will it grow back?" When superficially removed, moles can grow back, but it takes them quite a long time. "Yes," I reply, "come back in twenty or thirty years, and we'll flatten it again." When moles are excised, their return appearance is rare.

Large moles that cover a square inch or more of skin area will have to be excised, and more than likely will require skin grafting in the area. This means that a piece of skin is removed from behind the ear, or from the buttocks or legs, in order to place it on the mole removal site.

Skin tags are mole-like appendages—extra pieces of skin that hang like a mole, usually from armpit or neck. Skin tags do not become cancerous, but they can get irritated—as when they catch on clothing—and bleed. Grandma used to take a hair and tie it around the appendage to cause it to drop off. Today, we just take a scissors and snip the skin tag off. However, you'd better not make this a do-it-yourself project. Let your doctor handle skin tags.

You should know that moles are generally benign, that they can normally enlarge or grow hair, that they can also normally disappear and fade into the skin. Moles may develop a small stalk and fall off. Moles can be pink, brown, black, blue-black, or mottled in color. Moles can darken as a normal part of their life cycle.

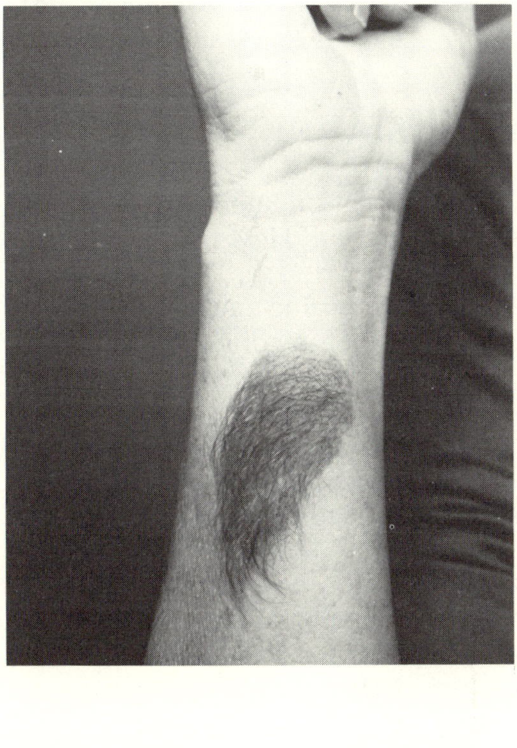

Hairy mole on forearm—needs to be surgically removed.

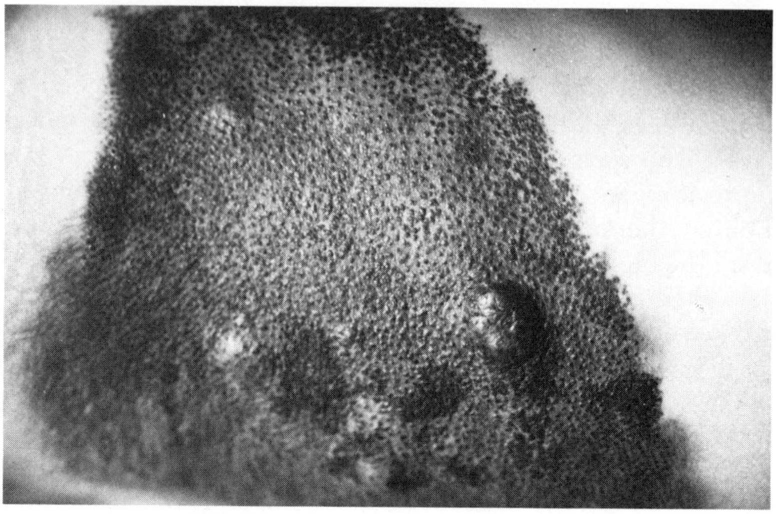

"Bathing suit" mole that developed melanoma (cancer).

But these changes are usually gradual and moderate. Any sudden, dramatic change in a mole can be cause for suspicion, as can bleeding or itching.

Five thousand people die of skin cancer annually in the United states. A sizeable percentage of these terminal cases start off with moles and become melanoma. Watch your moles, Mr. and Ms. Vigilante!

What to Watch for in Rashes

Rashes can be caused by external or internal factors. We will discuss rashes in more detail later on. However, just permit me to alert you to danger signs in a rash.

A rash is dangerous when it starts oozing and smelling.

A bad odor usually means that what might have been a passing rash has now become infected. Even an infected rash, if small in area—as on a finger—is unlikely to cause a major problem. Exception: Even if only one finger is infected, it could be harboring the *streptococcus*—which can be damaging to a vital organ, especially the kidney, where it can cause Bright's disease, or nephritis.

Poison ivy and the other common rashes (for which we will be providing you with home treatment methods later) are not dangerous unless they become impetigo—a bacterial infection of the skin. Strep is potentially more harmful than *staphylococcus*, even though most people react with more concern to the latter.

Chicken pox, if not scratched, usually causes no scars. Scratching causes a secondary infection, which is what causes the scars. Many of the so-called children's diseases are never diagnosed as such, because they do not cause the usual fever. The rash comes and goes, and you have had your measles.

The "adult" diseases are another matter. I am referring to skin rashes due to venereal disease. More about how to recognize the signs of these conditions later.

Meanwhile, treat a rash by not scratching it. Use soothing calamine lotion, cold water, and talcum powder. If the rash does not go away in a few days, or at least improve, phone your doctor. Talk to him or to the nurse, and see what they say. Your physician may want to give you an antihistamine to relieve the itch, especially if you are losing sleep. Lost sleep equals lost resistance and increased irritability. Your doctor may want to check the rash to spot infection, or to see if it may be contagious.

An inconvenient location of any rash should be treated professionally. A rash on the penis prohibiting sexual functioning, a rash on the eyelids affecting normal sight—these are you doctor's domain.

A woman came into my office with a rash on her eyelids. Her eyelids were so puffy that she could hardly see. She said she had stopped using mascara over a week ago, but this had not helped. As I made a note on the records, I noticed her rubbing her eyes with her hands. I suspected that the woman had a contact dermatitis—an irritation from some material she was using in her work.

I told her to put on cold compresses every hour on the hour, if possible. Cold compresses quiet swelling, because cold water constricts the blood vessels that supply the fluid to swelled areas. I gave this patient a prescription for an antihistamine pill, to reduce itching, and I gave an injection of cortisone (an anti- inflammatory drug) in the buttocks.

I also made some tests, and found that she was allergic to the photocopying equipment that she was using in her job.

Well, so much for skin problem highlights. We have touched on several conditions most briefly, but will now get into ways to prevent them, reduce them, and minimize them.

After that—on to skin health, vibrance, radiance, luster, and youthfulness.

Something Can be Done About Acne

Acne. For millions, the dirtiest four-letter word in the English language.

Beautiful girls and good-looking young men are transformed into social "lepers" by acne pocks and scars. Acne strikes the face most frequently, and there proclaims itself to the world.

Even its scientific name recognizes how disgusting its progressively deteriorating appearance can become: acne vulgaris.

Nobody ever died from acne, but many have described the disease as "a fate worse than death."

But: acne can be treated. Acne cannot be cured, but it can be prevented from becoming "progressively deteriorating."

This should cause some 80 percent of all adolescents to sit up and take notice, half of these as if their future depended on it. Maybe it does.

Many adults, too, get acne. Some adults are afflicted in their twenties and thirties, but acne can also strike people in their forties and fifties, affecting careers and human relationships.

The ostensible cause of acne is a hormone imbalance. Both men and women have hormones, so acne strikes both sexes. Acne erupts most frequently when the production of hormones is accelerating, during puberty—adolescence, that is. Some studies say that all adolescents have acne, but many have such mild cases that the symptoms are not easily seen.

You may think that you do not have acne and never had acne. Acne starts with blackheads. So think again.

The blackhead, or comedo, is created when excessive oil, produced by hormones, collects in a pore. A whitehead forms. The next phase brings pimples and cysts.

In this chapter, I am going to give you helpful advice on acne: controlling the condition, minimizing its visible effects, even reducing future attacks. I will also enumerate the do's and don'ts that can improve your good looks.

What Acne Really Is

Acne is not caused by diet. What you eat has no effect on acne. So go ahead, young man, or young lady, enjoy that candy bar. At least it won't show on your face.

If food does not aggravate acne, then what does cause acne, and what makes acne progress, persist, flare up?

When you think about causes, you need to think on several levels. You can say that oil, collecting in pores or oil gland openings, causes acne. You can then go to another level, and point to the hormones that cause excessive oil to be produced. And, if you want to go to a still deeper causative level and examine why the hormones behave abnormally, you can point to inherited tendencies, and to stress, worry, and anxiety.

When you want to treat acne, you think at one level. When you want to prevent or minimize acne, you need to think at another level.

The best place to start is with the start of acne.

Acne starts as a blackhead. The male sex hormone, testosterone, which females also have, causes the oil production that starts the disease known as acne. The oil may collect in a few pores, usually around the cheeks or nose, causing a few blackheads, which may last just a few weeks or a few months and then disappear, never to return again.

People whose blackheads disappear naturally do not realize how lucky they are. They have had acne in its initial phase. The

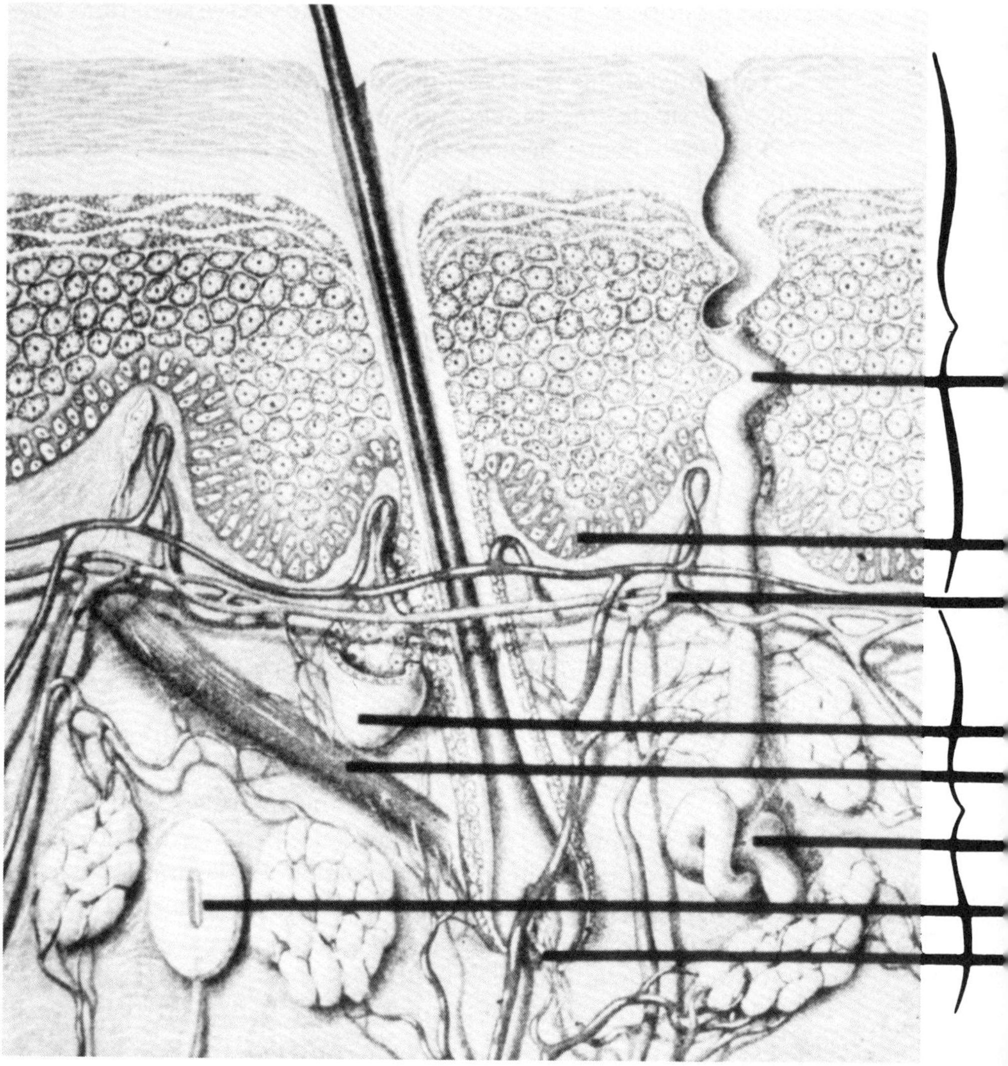

Cross section of normal skin.

acne could have gotten worse. It could have returned. This is the usual pattern. But when acne neither gets worse nor returns, these fortunate people never make the statistics. Add them to those who do, and the percentage of people that get acne may very well be 99 percent or even close to 100 percent.

Let's get a little more scientific.

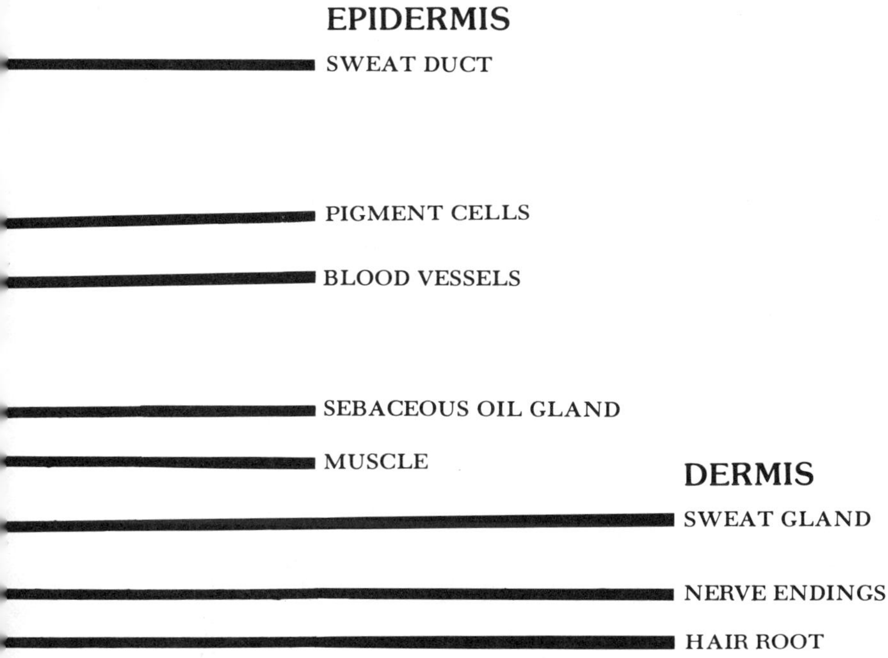

At the time of adolescence or emotional stress, the oil glands (sebaceous glands) of the skin enlarge. This enlargement is caused by increased activity of the endocrine glands that secrete hormones. The skin of the acne-prone person may react abnormally to those hormones, with changes that lead to the development of blackheads and pimples.

Often the openings of the ducts of large oil glands are visible as "pores" of the skin. Most of the oil formed by these glands reaches the surface of the skin. However, some of the material may be dammed back in the ducts of the large oil glands, where it produces blackheads and whiteheads. Some of the oily materials may break through the wall of the ducts and cause pimples and boils. In addition, this oily material may become infected, causing a greater amount of irritation to the surrounding skin.

If we call the blackhead low-grade acne, or grade one acne, then grade two acne is when the blackhead remains in the skin and becomes a pustule or pimple.

Grade three acne occurs when a deeper cyst forms. A cyst not only goes deeper than a blackhead or pimple, but erupts more insidiously as well, causing a severely marred complexion, and later, lesions and scars.

Acne starts as an oil-filled pore, a pore that has become blocked. Dirt does not create blackheads, as most people think. A blackhead is oxidized oil. The oil comes to the surface of the skin, air touches it, the oil oxidizes, and becomes black.

So soap and water do not help acne. Oily preparations, whether cleansers, suntan lotions, or other cosmetic products, can make matters worse. "Worse" means that grade one acne becomes grade two acne, and if not treated properly, grade two acne very quickly becomes grade three acne.

Acne strikes most of its victims on the face and neck alone. However, acne can attack the back and chest, as well as other areas of the body.

One of my patients, a male, had just been married. His bride knew of his body acne, but after just a few weeks it was wrecking their marital life. She found the sight and odor of his acne-ridden body so obnoxious, that even after he was successfully treated, the disease arrested, and some of the scars removed by an abrasive treatment, she still insisted on a divorce.

The patient had become extremely depressed, and even suicidal. Treatment may have saved his life, from that standpoint. Had he begun treatment earlier, he could have saved his marriage.

Acne has a terrible odor. It smells like fermented cheese. If acne covers extensive body areas, it permeates the place where the person lives. The odor of acne can be detected in some cases the minute the person walks into a room. Acne is decidedly unpleasant.

This newly-wed man was put in the hospital. Areas of his skin were frozen with liquid nitrogen: this is called cryosurgery. Cryosurgery is effective and relatively painless. The skin dries and peels, leaving new skin in its place. In some areas where there are deep lesions, repeated treatments are necessary.

The man was also given dermabrasion, a sandpapering-like treatment that is somewhat more painful than cryosurgery, extremely lengthy, and indeed, quite bloody. The afflicted bridegroom was also assisted by a plastic surgeon, who grafted new skin from unaffected parts of the patient's body to the more seriously scarred areas.

The acne sufferer became excited as he saw the changes in his body. He was more than 50 percent improved. He was released a happy man, and an easier man to look at, even though a bachelor again.

This was acne at its worst.

How to Control Acne

The usual case of acne is quite different.

The average patient comes into my office with a few blackheads. By simply using a blackhead remover, I quickly extract the potential troublemakers.

A blackhead remover is obtainable at most pharmacies, usually for under one dollar. It is worth many times its price to the incipient acne sufferer. The kind of blackhead remover that I prefer is made by LaCross. Other kinds of extractors just do not do as good a job.

You hold the LaCross instrument in your hand, place it over the blackhead, and push down. The blackhead just pops out. Then the pore returns to its normal size.

The longer the blackhead remains, the more distended the pore becomes, so the sooner you get after the blackhead, the better. Do not squeeze with the fingers. Use the blackhead remover.

If the condition has been present for some length of time, it can still be grade one acne, but additional steps may have to be taken to effect an improvement.

These additional steps include drying, peeling, special soaps, and over-the-counter lotions. Typical preparations are Fostril, Transact, and Sebanil (an astringent)—all over-the-counter preparations used after the patient washes. One may be tinted, another transparent. But all these products keep the skin dry and peeling.

These external preparations do not cause wrinkles, as many women fear. They cause only peeling, which is what we want to happen. We want to replace the ugly patches with new skin, which regenerates from below.

A critical time for women is just prior to the menstrual period. This is when the fluid is retained, and the oil in the pores increases. Many women have found that for a few days prior to their period, it is wise to use acne preparations. With men, there is no way to make such predictions.

The above treatment can ostensibly remove all visible signs of acne. But the acne-prone individual is not out of the woods. He or she must be a "vigilante," watching for the first sign of the return of those blackheads, and, of course, for the pimples.

Special note to teenagers: Waiting to "outgrow" your acne can be a serious mistake. Prompt treatment—even the simple treatment of removing the blackheads with the instrument described above, and applying the special after wash preparations—can prevent ugly pimples, boils, and cysts.

Acne is not "outgrown." Acne needs to be treated. Nor is acne a disease of dirt. Acne cannot be washed away. The blackness of a blackhead is not dirt, but is due to the oxidation of trapped oil.

The vigilant male student watches his skin more carefully prior to exams or important athletic or student activity events; so does the vigilant female student. The vigilant mature female watches her skin more carefully before menstrual periods. The vigilant mature male watches his skin during periods of special tension, anxiety, or economic stress.

As I said before, vigilance does not mean staying off chocolate. Let me explain.

Back in 1969, several doctors decided to test the widespread belief that chocolate is harmful in cases of acne. They enlisted the help of sixty-five volunteers. Thirty of these volunteers were adolescents attending a special acne clinic at Philadelphia's University Hospital. The sexual division among the volunteers was fourteen girls and sixteen boys. The thirty-five young adult male inmates of a local penal institution also volunteered.

Most of these sixty-five volunteers believed that chocolate was bad for acne. Some were sure that chocolate would be "disastrous" for their skins.

Before the test, the lesions on one side of the face were counted. Then the volunteers were given chocolate to eat— more chocolate than they would normally eat. What half of the subjects did not know was that they had been given "placebo" bars—harmless synthetic materials made to look and taste like chocolate bars.

The net result of the experiment was that those who ate the real chocolate showed no change in the condition of their acne as compared to those who ate the fake chocolate. There was no increase in the output of skin sebum among the chocolate eaters.

The conclusion by the doctors performing the experiment was that claims that high carbohydrate and high fat foods stimulate sebaceous secretion and adversely affect acne are unproved.

Teenagers, in case you would like to cheer these doctors, they are James E. Fulton, Gerd Plewig, and Albert M. Kligman, all dermatologists. But don't give chocolate a clean bill of health altogether. Why? For starters, ask your dentist.

Perhaps one quarter of grade one acne progresses to grade two acne. This is far more likely to happen where the person has been somewhat less than vigilant.

Preventing the More Advanced Stages of Acne

Many cases of acne will never have to see the inside of a dermatologist's office. These are the cases where the person has been aware of the need to watch his skin and take action, to keep his complexion acne-free.

This action can be personal action, taken without professional help. It means:

- Avoid oil-based cosmetics or greasing the skin. (No vanishing cream, no cold cream, no Noxzema, no moisturizers.)

- Use water-based or alcohol-based cosmetics. (Read the labels.)

- Get sunshine in moderation on your skin.

- Remove blackheads with the LaCross instrument.

- Apply the medications mentioned above after washing.

When a label does not indicate whether a product is water-based or alcohol-based (rather than oil-based), you can determine this by rubbing some of the liquid on a brown paper bag. Then turn the bag over. If the liquid produces a stain on the other side of the bag, the product is oil-based and should be avoided.

You can empty out or remove blackheads and whiteheads, but never use the fingers. If you squeeze with your fingers, you are squeezing in two directions. In effect, you are applying pressure at approximately 180 degrees, not on a complete circle, as with the blackhead remover. So the movement of the material is lateral, not vertical. The oil escapes to adjacent areas, widening the trouble spot.

Also, squeezing with the fingers is two-dimensional. The cyst or pimple can break underneath instead of on top. This causes a "foreign body" reaction under the skin when the oil is released there. Result: an aggravation of the condition both functionally and esthetically. The blackhead remover prevents both lateral and beneath-the-skin release, and the blackhead pops out.

Tests carried out by a medical team, where blackheads were removed from one side of the forehead and cheeks of patients but not the other side, showed that this procedure did indeed make a difference in preventing the development of inflamed lesions. You can bet that when the test was completed, those patients returned to "turn the other cheek."

This procedure, however, is rarely useful in the more advanced cases of cystic acne.

Treatment of Grade Three Acne

Your acne continues to worsen.

Why you? You have washed your face several times a day. You have been off chocolate, and even other sweets. You have been careful to squeeze blackheads and whiteheads whenever you spotted them.

Of course, by now you realize that these three most common deterrents are really not deterrents at all. Washing excessively can irritate rather than help. Diet has no effect on acne. And extracting, not squeezing, is the proper procedure for removing blackheads.

Even with proper procedure, acne can worsen. It can begin to take the form of surface blotches, pimples, and scars.

Why? The only cause behind the cause that we can come up with (besides genetically susceptible oil glands), is stress. Those ugly valleys and peaks are, in effect, a relief map of your anxieties.

We cannot change our genes. Our parents' genetic make-up determined our genes.

There is no salve to treat stress, and no block to impose to prevent its eruption on the skin you live in.

Stress is the villain in many diseases. The old-time family doctor knew this, and would frequently prescribe a trip to "get away from it all." Things move faster today. Time is money: double trouble. Opportunities to get away are harder to come by, and stress is more intense.

I am not going to advise you to try to avoid stress. Stress is not something one seeks out. Perhaps teaching patients to handle stress better would be a useful approach for doctors to take. There will be more on this in a later chapter.

Your acne is worse. It is getting out of hand—your hand. It

may not have been necessary to see your general practitioner or dermatologist up until now. But the time has surely come.

Let us examine some of the alternative treatments open to your doctor. His decision will be based on the needs of your skin.

The cyst of grade three acne is a space under the skin surrounded by a capsule of connective tissue. The bigger the cyst gets, the more space it occupies, and when the skin regresses back to normal—whether spontaneously or after infection—the bigger the scar the cyst will leave as a permanent mar to the complexion.

Louise, a sixteen-year-old high school girl, came to my office with acne—and with her mother. Louise's acne was a grade three case of neglect. Her mother was a grade one case of over-possessiveness. I don't know which was giving Louise more trouble.

Louise kept looking at the floor. She had gotten in the habit of looking down, to keep her face from being seen. Poor Louise, her very soul was scarred, too.

Louise said she had washed her face frequently under her mother's orders, and used her Noxzema regularly. "I don't eat chocolate, and I have been doing everything I am supposed to do," she offered in her own defense.

"Noxzema is not right for acne," I explained.

Louise was startled. She looked at her mother, and her flaming nostrils said, "See, I told you so."

"It says on the jar to use Noxzema for acne," her mother replied. Now *she* was on the defensive.

"Noxzema is an oil-based preparation. No oil-based preparation will help acne. It just compounds the problem, which is *oil*."

Louise and her mother looked at each other.

"What do you use on your scalp?" I asked Louise, hoping to ease the tention. This question made matters still worse. Mother had recommended another product— again oil-based.

I gave Louise the names of one or two over-the- counter preparations that she should use for her face, and another for her scalp. I showed her how to use a blackhead remover. I then gave her a prescription for an antibiotic.

Tetracycline is an effective antibiotic for acne. The success of tetracycline in relieving acne symptoms is thought to be related to the fat metabolism of skin bacteria rather than to specific antibacterial properties of the drug. Yes, tetracycline kills germs and halts infection, but more important, it gets into the oily areas and changes their structure so that bacteria cannot multiply there.

The dosage of tetracycline varies from one to four capsules a day, which must be spaced out so that the pills are not taken with meals. For Louise, I prescribed an initially large dose to be taken for the first two weeks, followed by a smaller maintenance dose. Light dosages of antibiotics are quite effective in treating acne. In fact, the antibiotic can be taken over a period of years without any harmful effects. The price of tetracycline is quite low, sometimes running under five cents a capsule.

Tetracycline has very few contra-indications or possible harmful side effects. A rash or gastric upset is rare. Tetracycline is not be taken by pregnant women, or while breast feeding. The antibiotic can get into the teeth of the fetus or infant and cause stains. Also, tetracycline is not to be taken by women who are prone to vaginal yeast infections. Such infections can be made worse by antibiotics.

Some antibiotics are sun-sensitizers. If you are out in the sun a good portion of the day, or if you live in Florida, Hawaii, or a subtropical area, your physician will not prescribe an antibiotic that causes unfavorable reactions in strong sunshine.

Do not expect immediate results from antibiotics. They take time to work, at least as far as visible improvement goes. Even a successful antibiotic treatment might take a month to "show."

I explained this fact to Louise. I also told her that chocolate might not be the best thing for her to eat, but it would have no effect on her acne.

"Eat and drink what you want. Go yourself to the pharmacy to buy this instrument," I directed, holding up the blackhead remover. "Then use it yourself. If Mother does it for you, it might hurt too much."

I think Louise's mother began to get the message. She knew I was encouraging Louise to be more self-reliant in her own treatment. This would reduce mother-daughter friction. Less friction, possibly less acne.

There is a positive aspect to this, too. Many patients get a psychological gratification out of watching the blackhead come out. More pleasure, possibly less acne.

Louise came back in two weeks for a checkup. She no longer looked down. She looked me straight in the face, and her own face wore a great big smile. Louise still had some blackheads, some cysts. But her skin was not oily; it was dry. It was responding. "No need for our going into any other type of treatment," I assured her. "Keep up the good work." I smiled, too, as she left, our mutual smiles permitting to remain unspoken the words "Mother stayed home."

New Approaches to Acne: Vitamin A Acid Therapy and Benzoyl-Peroxide

Vitamin A helps to improve the skin in some acne cases. The required amounts of Vitamin A (400,000 units a day), taken internally, would be toxic for most people. They would probably lose their hair, develop eye problems, and possibly develop tumor-like lumps in the brain.

So Vitamin A is placed directly on the skin. One available product is Retin-A, retinoic acid or Vitamin A acid. Retin-A is a prescription drug, available either in liquid gel or foil-covered saturated swabs.

One Retin-A swab per day is the usual application. Be prepared for the acne to get worse before it gets better. The acid causes peeling, and this action is apparently unrelated to the medication's physiologic function as a vitamin. After the peeling, the blackheads dry up and surface, new blackheads do not form as readily, and cysts become permeable, causing irritants to leak out.

Sometimes Retin-A causes temporary redness, burning, and stinging, in which case the frequency can be adjusted or the treatment discontinued temporarily. Also, exposure to bright sunlight for any lengthy periods can cause burning faster than usual. Keep Retin-A away from the eyes, eyelids, nostrils, and corners of the mouth.

In a recent clinical test, 38.8 percent of the acne patients treated with Retin-A showed an excellent result (measured as a

75 percent or greater acne reduction). The closest runner-up was benzoyl peroxide, with 4.1 percent. Also, 37.8 percent treated with Retin-A showed a good result (measured as a 50 percent to 74 percent acne reduction). The closest runner-up again was benzoyl peroxide, with 26.5 percent of the users showing good results.

I consider Retin-A and benzoyl peroxide, also a prescription drug, the two most promising developments in the treatment of acne. They should be reserved for patients who do not do well with over-the-counter preparations. Commonly sold commercial names are Desquamex, Panoxyl, and Benoxyl: all benzoyl peroxide products.

Benzoyl peroxide is a drying preparation that adds oxygen to the skin to help healing. Benzoyl peroxide preparations far surpass in effectiveness the older preparations, which were combinations of sulphur, salycilic acid, and other drying ingredients.

Retin-A acts beneficially largely as an irritant. Benzoyl peroxide acts beneficially by adding healing oxygen to the skin. In sunny climes, the choice should be benzoyl peroxide.

A few miscellaneous notes.

Women with acne will note premenstrual flare-ups. These can be avoided by taking diuretics a few days before the expected onset of menstruation. Diuretics help to eliminate the fluids that accumulate prior to the period. The acne gets worse, because the top layers of the skin get soggy. Diuretics taken five or six days before the period cause increased urination and a lessening in this fluid buildup. Consider these five or six days as a maximum period. Prolonged use can cause depletion of potassium with resulting muscle weakness.

If you have acne, look for dandruff. Dandruff and acne are basically the same conditions. The scalp oil gland produces either an oily or dry scale. Like acne, the dandruff scales are caused by hormones, made worse by stress. If you don't treat dandruff with an anti-dandruff shampoo, you are only partially treating acne.

Sunshine helps acne—if you do not use an oil-based preparation. Use an alcohol preparation like Pre-Sun or Pabafilm. (See the chapter on the sun, pages 72-91.)

When inquiring at the pharmacy regarding non-oil-based acne preparations, men will want to ask for the transparent varieties, as opposed to the tinted preparation that women frequently prefer.

Sometimes we treat acne with X-rays, sometimes with cortisone, but rarely. Cryosurgery is excellent for acne. We use this treatment more and more.

The Emotional Factor in Acne

We have already discussed the fact that stress is a primary cause of acne. Let's face up to it. Suppressing that understanding will not fool your skin.

First, I want to repeat that the physiological cause of acne is a hormone increase. The hormone increase affects the oil glands: more oil is produced by the glands. This is the most likely to occur in individuals between the ages of thirteen to sixteen and twenty-five to thirty-five. As the oil in the skin contacts the air, it is oxidized, and forms a blackhead. The blackhead is hard and dense. The blackhead prevents the deeper oil from coming out. So the oil collects. Cysts form.

We understand this. But now we need to understand what causes the hormone production to increase.

Sometimes the mere advent of puberty stimulates hormone production. But why doesn't puberty bring acne to everybody? The answer seems to reside in individual variation in tolerance to stress. Hormone balance is affected by stress.

For a bridge girder or roof rafter, stress is the amount of physical load it must carry. For a human being, stress is the amount of emotional load he or she must carry.

What is an emotional load? Mother can be an emotional load to a child seeking to be its own person. So can Father. Boyfriend or girlfriend can be an emotional load. And school. And peer activities.

The chain reaction may not be totally understood. What exactly is the link between hormone production and the upcoming final exam, the prom, the need to engineer Dad's permission? We don't really know. We know that stress causes tension, that this tension can be measured with biofeedback devices as it affects tiny musculature, that these effects go all the way to vital organs.

I don't mind confessing that I get a great deal of satisfaction out of relieving stress in my acne patients in any way I can. You may have detected the glee with which I helped Louise get out from under the duress her mother was heaping on her, or the pleasure it gives me to tell a patient to go ahead and eat chocolate. These factors relieve stress and insure patient cooperation.

I am not against mothers, or in favor of chocolate, but as a dermatologist I am aware of the initial emotional cause behind the physical effects that lead to skin conditions like acne.

The reason twenty-five to thirty-five is a critical age bracket for persons susceptible to acne is that the hormones react on oil at this stage in life the same way that they react at puberty. Also, the skin has dried out, so oil cosmetics are being used more. Some women are afraid that this late acne signals the change of life. It doesn't. Nor is the skin affected by a change of lovers. Sexual activity plays no role in acne, unless those sexual relationships are causing stress.

Your awareness of emotional impact on acne is just as important as my awareness. Reading this page can conceivably prevent acne. If you have incipient acne, perhaps evidenced by a few blackheads, your understanding that stress can be the trigger for a flare-up can defuse it.

Come tension time, you might "face up" to the need to be more philosophical, more tolerant, more patient, more confident— just knowing that the attractiveness of your face is at stake, and that if you don't "cool it," your skin will erupt with the heat of your emotions.

I believe that there must be at least dermatological validity to what some say is the Eleventh Commandment: "Thou shalt not sweat it."

Acne sufferers are the most insecure people on earth— socially, sexually, and economically. Just by giving the acne patient a little hope that some improvement can be made in a short time, even two or three weeks, I give these people an emotional boost.

Acne scars the psyche as well as the skin. A person sees in the acne not a short-term sentence, but condemnation for life. If you are not an acne sufferer, it is difficult for you to feel this torment.

Yet, this suffering can all be avoided. Treated in time, acne is not a life sentence.

I wish I could stand on a streetcorner and shout about the

advisability of extracting blackheads and the availability of helpful, non-oily, over-the-counter preparations. "Hey, you. Blackheads on the upper cheeks. Extract them tonight. Then use Fostril, Transact, or Sebanil." Of course, I cannot do this; but it would certainly reach some of those countless thousands of marred-for-life people who look in the mirror daily and agonize, "Why didn't somebody tell me?"

A patient comes into my office with a half-dozen blackheads. Man, woman, or child, the patient says, "I hate to bother you, Doctor."

"Bother?" I reply, "I love to see patients like this. In a few minutes of treatment and explanation, I can save a psyche."

Psoriasis Need be no Heartbreak

While enjoying my hobby—photography—I have captured on film characteristics of the surface of planet earth that compare remarkably closely with characteristics of the surface of the human body. Volcanos look strikingly like skin eruptions. Dried-up lake beds have cracks like over-dry skin. There is hardly a skin condition known to man that mother earth does not have also—except one.

Nowhere on earth have I been able to photograph a condition that compares with psoriasis.

Psoriasis is a common condition among humans. It affects one out of every fifty persons in the United States, showing no preference for sex or color.

Psoriasis is a skin condition that shows up as thick, reddish, silvery-scaled patches. It may be confined to one or two small, local areas, or it may cover large areas of the body, and occasionally the entire body.

More commonly, psoriasis appears on the elbows, knees, scalp, and trunk areas. Psoriasis can also appear under the arms, on the head of the penis, or in the groin.

'How can I live this down?"

"I'm staying home—I'm ashamed to be seen."

"They'll think I have leprosy."

Reactions like these cause psoriasis to be known as the "heartbreak" skin disease.

Believe me, this epithet is not deserved. Psoriasis responds to treatment. There need be no heartbreak. The television commercials exploiting that word do a disservice to psoriasis patients. The word "heartbreak" depresses them unnecessarily, makes psoriasis sound like an irreversible tragedy. Actually, psoriasis is reversible, in fact fairly speedily reversible, and certainly no tragedy.

Psoriasis cannot be cured permanently. But attacks of psoriasis can be treated successfully. These treatments are usually effective in a matter of days, but severe cases might take weeks to subside.

For most people, relief from further attacks of psoriasis may last only several weeks, but for lucky ones the respite can be years.

What causes psoriasis? Why do some people get the disease frequently, and others not at all? We do not yet know the answers, but we do have a few clues. And we do have a few effective treatments for psoriasis.

In this chapter we will describe these methods of treatment for psoriasis at various locations and of various degrees of severity, and we will discuss ways to lessen the chance of developing this skin disease, especially if you are psoriasis-prone.

Is Psoriasis Dangerous?

The greatest pain that psoriasis creates is emotional. Psoriatic patients become distressed by their appearance. There is certainly nothing pretty about the scaly patches. The borders are clearly marked.

A teenaged girl with psoriasis on her elbows will wear a long- sleeved blouse or dress no matter how warm the weather. A man with psoriasis on his genitals will abstain from sex. Any person with psoriasis of the scalp will find the shedding of large amounts of silver, white, or grey scales a source of social embarrassment.

What appears to be happening in psoriasis cases is an acceleration in the growth of skin cells. The normal life of an outer skin cell is twenty-five to thirty days. In psoriasis, the time from the formation of the skin cell to the time of its shedding is accelerated to a period of four to five days.

This out-of-control cell growth makes psoriasis a third cousin to cancer. But there the similiarity stops. Psoriasis is not malignant. It is relatively harmless. And it is reversible.

The reversing process can be spontaneous, or the result of treatment. Psoriasis leaves no scars, and the skin returns to a normal, healthy appearance. How long the skin remains healthy before the next attack is subject to wide variation.

I have personally never known of anybody who died from psoriasis. Psoriasis is not considered fatal. It is certainly not contagious.

This is not to say there have not been psoriatic deaths in the record. The greatest threat is when psoriasis covers the entire body. The flow of blood to the skin may then nearly double, and the resulting strain on the heart can cause heart failure.

Some 10 percent of psoriatics get psoriatic arthropathy—a very painful form of the disease that causes arthritic symptoms, even in thirty year olds, and can lead to severe damage in the hands and feet in one's most productive years.

A siege of not-so-bad psoriasis can become so bad as to necessitate hospitalization.

When severe flare-ups of psoriasis occur, there can be a painful reddening over large areas of the body. The skin can crack around joints. Lesions start as small, drop-like breaks in the skin all over the areas affected, and can spread to cover the whole skin.

This is acute psoriasis. It causes chills, severe discomfort, and the shedding of large amounts of scaling skin. I usually recommend that such a patient be hospitalized, as the treatment is quite intensive. This extreme form of the disease is known as erythroderma psoriaticum, or exfoliative psoriasis.

Such cases are rare. The more common situation by far is when psoriasis is confined to a small area of the body. Here comes such a patient now.

The Elbows—Favorite Location of Psoriasis

Miss L.W., age twenty, is a secretary, but could pass for a model. She is quite attractive and chic. Today Miss L. W. is wearing long sleeves. In these days of abbreviated styles, long sleeves on a warm day, worn by an attractive girl, may spell elbow psoriasis.

I look at Miss L. W.'s nails. She has tiny holes in them, which she has not been able to camouflage with nail polish. The holes appear as cross-gidings, or small pits. Miss L. W. pulls her hand away. "Aren't they disgraceful? But they're not why I'm here."

'Yes, they are," I reply. "They are connected with your elbow condition."

Miss L. W. gives me that how-did-you-know look, as she pulls up her sleeves and exhibits her plaqued elbows.

I examine her elbows. I will treat them with bland (non-burning, non-irritating) creams or ointments, such as Vaseline or cold creams containing menthol to cool the skin. Here is a thicker patch, so I will suggest Estar Gel.

Estar Gel is a purified tar in a watery, alcoholic gel form. Estar Gel is similar to Tegrin, the most advertised antipsoriatic preparation. Tegrin contains a tar extract, and allantoin to help heal the skin, but is not as effective as Estar Gel. Any kind of tar soap, tar ointment, or tar lotion is helpful for psoriasis. Tar, for

Typical psoriasis of the elbow.

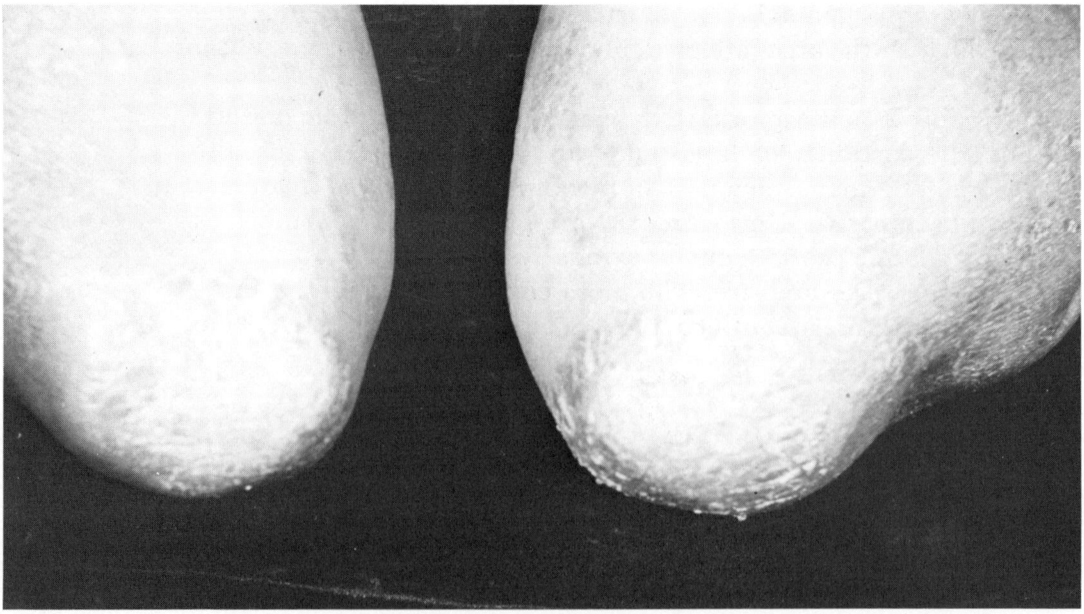

some reason that we do not fully understand, stops cells from multiplying. Since the abnormally rapid multiplying of cells is the reason for psoriasis, tar brings about a noticeable improvement.

While applying the Estar Gel to Miss L.W.'s elbows, I explain another characteristic of tar products.

"Roll up your sleeves during lunch hour, and get some sun on your elbows. Sun alone helps, but this product increases the benefits of sun on your elbows. You do not need a prescription for Tegrin. Apply it two or three times a day."

When Miss L. W. returned in a few days, the patches on her elbows were reduced in size and less discolored. In a week, her psoriasis was gone, though not all psoriasis clears that fast.

Pitted nails are not restored that fast. Most physicians will not treat the nails—an injection of cortisone being about the only course available and too drastic a measure to take for purely cosmetic reasons. In time, the nails frequently normalize—until the next attack.

Most psoriatic patients who come to me have already tried one or more of the fifteen over-the-counter preparations available to them. In fact, there used to be even more preparations available, but now ammoniated mercury has been removed from the market by the Federal Drug Administration as not safe. However, these drugstore items are frequenty not properly applied.

If you have a thick scale, you need to remove it before applying the preparation. This you do by washing the area thoroughly, and using a scrubbing brush to remove the loose skin. Then apply the ointment to the scale.

It is always advisable to see your dermatologist or physician before beginning self-treatment. It may be that he will advise a stronger course of action in your case, such as cortisone.

Cortisone is a powerful drug. It has a pronounced effect on psoriasis. Stubborn cases of psoriasis subside with surprising rapidity when treated with cortisone. Again, cortisone does not bring about a permanent cure of psoriatic conditions.

When bland ointments and tar preparations do not improve psoriasis of the elbows, cortisone is employed. The elbows (the most common locale for psoriasis) usually respond quite well to treatment, but the condition may recur at the elbow sites within weeks, months, or years.

How to Judge the Severity of Psoriasis

It has been jokingly said that there is an economic recession if *he* is out of work, but an economic depression if *we* are out of work.

The severity of psoriasis is also faced with a dual set of standards, one used when the physician is doing the evaluation, the second when the patient is judging it.

Back in 1970, a survey on psoriasis was made by a team at the Dartmouth Medical School. A number of symptoms and features connected with the disease were listed, and a sampling of doctors was asked to rate these factors as to their importance in contributing to the severity or mildness of a case of psoriasis. Their patients were given the same questionnaire.

When the doctors' replies were compared to the patients', it became apparent that doctor and patient had two widely different ways of judging the severity of the disease.

The physicians rated "shivering" as the symptom of psoriasis that reflected the greatest severity. The patients, however, ranked "shivering" as one of the least important symptoms, and instead rated "embarrassment over appearance" as the main indicator of the severity of psoriasis.

While the physicians rated fever as among the top danger signs of psoriasis, patients rated fever as the last symptom they would think important, and instead listed scales found in the bedding as the danger sign.

About the only vital factor that both patient and physician agreed on was when the entire body surface was affected by psoriasis.

Enlargement of an old patch of psoriasis causes many patients to expect that they are in for a psoriatic siege, whereas physicians look at this enlargement as pretty much par for the course. Scales in the clothing have a way of striking fear in the hearts of the wearers, but here again, physicians are less interested in this social condition and more interested in such factors as loss of hair or fingernails, interference with sleep, and the involvement of new areas of the body, including the advent of other types of psoriatic symptoms, such as arthritic swelling or pains in the joints.

How to Treat Serious Psoriasis

When a case of psoriasis appears serious enough to the physician to warrant "strong medicine," that medicine will probably be cortisone.

Cortisone is very effective against psoriasis. It is a prescription drug. Cortisone is available in cream (like cold cream or vanishing cream), ointments (which lubricate like vaseline), or in watery solutions or lotions for hairy areas. Some special forms of the drug such as cortisone tape are also now available. Cortisone may be injected directly into the skin. Sometimes this is painful, but it is not as bad as it sounds. The cortisone cream, ointment, solution, or lotion is applied directly to the affected skin, usually after a bath or shower or warm compress. This previous moistening of the skin permits the cortisone to reach deeper into the skin and do its job better.

When cortisone is injected into the bone or blood system, as is done when the drug is used to treat arthritis and other conditions, there is a tolerance limit of which physicians must be aware. However, when cortisone is applied on the skin, there are only a few contraindications to watch out for. The most prominent of these are when cortisone is applied under the armpits or in the groin area. Here, care must be used, as there could be a thinning of the skin if the cortisone is used for prolonged periods.

One way to decrease the period of cortisone use is to cover the area on which it has been applied with common kitchen plastic wrap, like Saran Wrap. Saran Wrap has the same effect as that warm compress or bath. It enables the cortisone to do the work better.

When you put cortisone on the skin, it lies there. But if you cover that area with Saran Wrap, Magic Wrap, or other plastic wrap—if on the foot, like a bootie; if on the abdominal area, taped down; if on the wrist, like a glove—the temperature and humidity of the skin increase at the covered area, and this permits the cortisone to penetrate deeper and to clear up the psoriasis faster. Cortisone is usually applied three or four times a day—but once is usually enough!

Whether your are treating the common elbow psoriasis or

other skin areas, if a cortisone cream or ointment is prescribed by your physician, inquire about some of the newer forms of cortisone and the tachyphylaxis approach to treatment. Use plastic wrap around your cortisone medication, to increase its penetration and speed the relief.

Psoriasis of the Penis

A thirty-year-old man came to my office. He had thought he had a veneral disease, but his physician diagnosed the condition as psoriasis and referred him to me.

This patient was a swinging bachelor type.

He was thoroughly distraught. His penis was useless, except to urinate. An emotional disaster.

"Do you use condoms?" I asked.

'Sometimes. Why do you ask? My doc says it's not VD."

"It's not VD. It's psoriasis, a skin disease," I replied as I wrote a cortisone cream prescription. "This medication will work faster if, after you apply it on the penis, you wear a condom."

He nodded, relieved.

He was free of his psoriasis attack in five days. And back to swinging.

Psoriasis is recurrent. It is never cured. Sometimes the period of reoccurence is quite long, long enough for the patient to think that he is cured.

On the other hand, some patients are visited by psoriasis every few weeks. Where a patient is psoriasis-prone, the disease can pop up in a number of locations, but most psoriasis patients have "favorite" places. If the elbows are number one, the penis, for males, is number two.

Psoriasis is not something people talk about. "Hey, I have psoriasis on my penis." But psoriasis is quite prevalent. Many people with psoriasis are silent about it, in fact, never even seek treatment. It is estimated that 75 percent of the psoriatics hide their affliction, never seek treatment, and suffer in silence. You can bet your pants most sufferers from psoriasis of the penis keep mum about their condition.

The sun, as a curative agent, is more applicable to the elbows than to the penis. But where sunbaths cannot be taken without risk of arrest for exposure, there is always the ultra-violet lamp.

Ultra-violet light should be used sparingly, though, as you can easily go from one skin problem—psoriasis—to another: acute burn. Never use the lamp in a position where you can fall asleep. A few short sunlamp treatments are better than one longer one.

Causes of Psoriasis

When we talk about skin cell growth increasing at a much faster than normal rate, we are talking about a metabolic change. This metabolic change can stop as fast as it starts.

In World War II, prisoners confined in German concentration camps got rid of their repeated attacks of psoriasis. Apparently, the starvation and the reduction of vitamins and minerals in the prison fare slowed down the body's metabolism. The change in metabolism was the key to the disappearance of the psoriasis.

Psoriasis is less common in skinny people, who usually have a naturally higher metabolic rate than their chubbier friends.

We can call metabolism a clue, but that's about all. Eventually, a cure may be found for psoriasis that may very well exploit this metabolic factor.

There is also an emotional factor in psoriasis. Many women get psoriasis before a menstrual period. Brides frequently get attacks before the wedding, reinforcing the "heartbreak" reputation of psoriasis.

Men commonly get outbreaks of psoriasis when they suffer a loss of job or a business setback, or when their emotional stance is shaken in love affairs, or by marital failure.

We do not really understand the mechanisms involved in the inception of psoriasis. The disease seems to lie in wait, so to speak, as a latent condition among psoriasis-prone people, and then flares up when there is emotional irritation.

Rose T., a forty-five-year-old housewife, struck me as a very emotional woman when I treated a mild case of psoriasis on her hands. She had family problems, and was very anxious to ventilate them to me.

The psoriasis responded to treatment, but then returned, worse than it was before. This happened several times. Each time, Rose continued to share her family problems with me, and I got the impression that these, too, were getting worse and worse.

This went on for months. Rose became very depressed, and was using tranquilizers, which of course dulled her feelings, but did nothing for her skin.

Pretty soon the psoriasis was so widespread that Rose would have to be hospitalized if I did not take some drastic action. Cortisone injections seemed to be called for. The drug was injected into Roses' bloodstream, via the buttocks, and in ten days her psoriasis had disappeared.

This seemed to boost Rose's morale. She got off the tranquilizers, and was able to cope with her family problems successfully.

Psoriasis can also flare up with physical irritation. Men who use certain tools; athletes who hold bowling balls, raquets, or clubs; women whose occupations create friction such as on the knees or elbows—all can be subject to these psoriasis flare-ups at the point of irritation.

Another clue lies in the way psoriasis acts toward sunlight. First, psoriasis seldom strikes areas that are exposed to sunlight. Facial psoriasis, for instance, is rare. Second, the condition responds favorably when affected areas are exposed to the direct rays of the sun.

At the present time, we cannot draw any conclusions from these clues. We base our treatments of psoriasis on them, but we cannot yet formulate a hypothesis that explains the cause-effect relationship behind psoriasis.

Nor does it help to know from the statistics that a genetic component also appears to be a factor in psoriasis. A large percentage of the descendants of psoriatics are afflicted with the disease sooner or later. But that does not mean every offspring of psoriatic parents will eventually have psoriasis.

There is no blood test for psoriasis. Susceptibility can frequently be detected by examining the skin around an irritation. The edges of the skin around the irritation may reveal the tiny flaking of psoriasis. Without such a medical test, diagnosis falls entirely on the physician's observation of the skin lesion, backed up with a laboratory's microscopic study of cells from the lesion.

No test.

No known cause.

No total cure.

Psoriasis may be one of the "heartbreaks" of science.

Psoriasis of the Scalp

Psoriasis often affects the scalp. When this happens, the patient at first thinks he has dandruff. Psoriasis is scaly, crusted, and flaky, and creates snowstorm effects on the collars and shoulders of clothing, just like dandruff.

However, there are serious differences between dandruff and psoriasis. Psoriasis of the scalp may cause a foul smell. And often the scales are thick, like mica.

Once the problem is identified as psoriasis, the patient needs to use a tar-based shampoo. Sebutone shampoo is one of these. Again, the tar acts to slow down the runaway cell growth.

After each shampoo, psoriatics can use a special solution like "P&S" solution. The "P" stands for phenol and the "S" for saline. This is an over-the-counter product. The phenol is an irritant to the skin that acts to support the effects of the tar.

Cortisone cream preparations are also effective on scalp psoriasis, but usually these are sticky, and so are rather messy to use. I seldom recommend them. Instead, I prefer a cortisone liquid or solution.

Again, the solution works better if you use a plastic shower cap after applying it. The shower cap helps the cortisone liquid to penetrate deeper into the scalp. You can sleep with the shower cap on for a few hours, or all night long. Result: faster relief from the annoying symptoms of scalp psoriasis.

A television newscaster in a large city—let's call him George L.—discovered his psoriasis before a broadcast when a prop man gave him a routine brush-off.

"You got some dandruff," said the prop man.

But George L. was never troubled with dandruff. That night, he gave himself a good shampoo. While drying his hair, he noticed discolored areas of his scalp. His physician told him the bad news—psoriasis.

George L. decided to have his hair dyed in order to better screen out the psoriasis patches on his scalp from possible view of his television audience. But they were still visible, as was the continuing "blizzard" of greyish-white scales.

When George L. came to my office, he told me this tale of woe, and I prescribed a steroid solution in the cortisone family. He agreed to wear a shower cap—*after* he went off the air and went home to bed. In ten days, the patches were gone.

The psoriasis was not gone for good, though. Every three or four weeks the signs reappeared. George L. would then apply the solution, wear the cap in bed, and in a few days the patches would disappear.

I had explained the stress factor to George L. His first attack occurred at election time, when he was being subjected to a tremendous amount of political pressure. George L. later told me that he would be especially observant of his scalp whenever "things got tight," and he found that his psoriasis seemed to creep back at these very times.

Anal Psoriasis

A bank vice president came to see me. I asked him to be seated, but he said he preferred to stand.

I soon understand why.

He told me where his complaint was, and I examined the area. He had a ring around his anus. It was psoriasis, even though it did not have the scales of psoriasis. In this part of the body, the moisture present prevents the scaling. This patient also had an irritation rash.

I asked the bank officer what he had been doing for the psoriasis. He listed a dozen over-the-counter and prescription preparations that he had been applying. These preparations had really added to his problem by causing what we call contact dermatitis. The man was allergic to several substances he was using. Foreign substances kept on the skin continuously can cause an irritation that compounds the original problem.

Skin preparations need to be quickly effective so that constant use is avoided. The banker was using a trial and error method. He tried one drug after another, seldom giving any one product time to be effective, and as a result had actually increased the irritation in the anal area. Now it was so painful that he could not sit down.

Can you imagine the kind of heartbreak this can mean to a bank officer?

I stopped all of this patient's self-applied medications. I instructed him to use only cold compresses for one week. When he returned, the rash was gone. His severe discomfort was gone. He could sit down.

We had the contact dermatitis beaten; now we went to work on the psoriasis.

I gave him a steroid cortisone cream to apply, and in a few days the psoriasis had disappeared.

Anal psoriasis knows no sexual discrimination. It can be temporarily conquered, but not permanently cured. Men or women get anal psoriasis, especially when they sit for long periods of time, or engage frequently in a physical activity that causes irritation around the thighs and buttocks. Again, emotional stress can also be a causative factor.

Psoriasis of the Hands or Feet

Because psoriasis is frequently triggered by irritation, many jobs involve this type of occupational hazard.

A mechanic who has a wrench in his hand a good part of the day is a candidate for psoriasis of the hand.

A fireman who wears boots a good deal can develop psoriasis of the feet due to the irritation of this heavy covering.

A hotel maid who must get down on her knees to clean the bathtubs can develop psoriasis of the knees.

All three of these psoriasis cases would require the cortisone ointment, and therapeutic results could be hastened by covering the affected area with a plastic covering at night.

A typical case of psoriasis of the hands was Frank P., who worked for a car repair shop. He was thirty-five years old, and married. Frank's wife accompanied him to my office, because the sight of Frank's hand was so frightening that she thought she could catch whatever he had, or that maybe the kids could catch it.

I assured her that Frank had psoriasis, and that it was not in the least contagious. The couple was so relieved that they started to walk out of the office, and I had to remind Frank that he was still suffering from psoriasis, but that his condition could be relieved in a few weeks.

"If you do not treat psoriasis, your wife will not get it from you, but *you* could get it from you. Untreated, the psoriasis could spread to larger areas of your hand, and the lesions could become deeper. You risk infection. Your hand might get fissures—thick cracks in the skin. Then it won't be just ugly to look at. It will hurt just to open your fingers."

Frank and his wife sat back down, and I wrote out a prescription for cortisone ointment. I told Frank that he needed a plastic glove, to cover the medicated hand at night to hasten results. "Borrow one from your wife," I suggested, and then turning to her, I repeated, "Mrs. P., it's not catching. You can wear that glove yourself again."

'I'll throw it out anyhow," she assured me, and they left.

Tar, cortisone. This has been the treatment story for psoriasis for a century. There have been some detours along the way.

In the 1880s tar was upstaged for a while by a remedy called chrysarobin. Chrysarobin grew steadily in favor with the medical profession then, as it was useful in a number of chronic skin diseases. However, as the use of chrysarobin continued, it was found to cause on occasion a violent contact dermatitis that was worse than the disease for which the medication was applied. Furthermore, just one application of the drug permanently stained clothing. Chrysarobin went through many combinations with other substances before it was relegated to medical annals, and tar products resumed their starring psoriatic role.

While researchers are still struggling to come up with answers that might lead to new avenues of psoriasis treatment, we must continue to resort to the "tried and true." This limits treatment of psoriasis to the tar-based and cortisone products, with a possible dash of sunlight, and a stress-relieving pat on the shoulder.

The treatment is the same for elbows, penis, anus, hands, feet, and other localized patches of psoriasis.

But add them all together, and the story becomes different.

When Psoriasis Attacks all of the Skin You Live in

A Filipino man, sixty-five years old, was referred to me by an intern of a hospital emergency room because of a "severe sunburn." I looked at the patient. He had psoriasis with exfoliation (peeling) over his entire body.

The patient was very uncomfortable. He was losing a lot of fluid through the skin, as he would with a severe burn. Through questioning him, I found that he had psoriasis on various parts of his body, and he treated it himself, first with one drugstore salve and then another.

I placed the man in the hospital. There is no way to treat such a total case of psoriasis as an outpatient. Intravenous fluids were provided to replace what his body had lost. He was also given special baths. Bath therapy is an old treatment for psoriasis, and it will probably be around for a long time to come.

Tar liquid—just a few drops—is placed in the bath water. It is soothing, and tends to cause a slowdown of the rapid cell growth that is psoriasis.

In three days, the redness of my elderly patient had quieted down, and we began treatment with a light box. Ultra-violet light of the sun is curative, and can be duplicated by special artificial light sources.

It took three weeks of hospitalization, but when the man left, he had healthy skin. He was advised to see his doctor any time local patches reappeared.

This treatment by tar and ultra-violet light is the accepted one for total body psoriasis. The treatment is frequently supplemented with cortisone and dressings at night.

How to Tell Whether You Have Psoriasis

Many skin conditions show characteristics quite like psoriasis. I was not surprised at the intern's mistaken diagnosis in

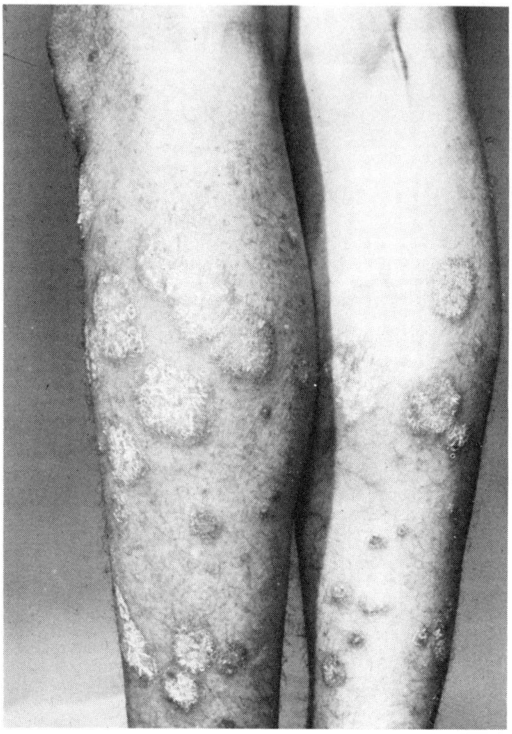

Psoriasis on legs.

the above case. More experienced doctors have been fooled. Some forms of eruptions due to eczema resemble psoriasis. Some fungal infections of the fingernails appear to be psoriasis, as does a skin disease called seborrheic dermatitis.

If you have a scaling of the skin that you think might be psoriasis, you might perform the following test yourself while awaiting the appointment date with your physician: scratch the skin lightly with your fingernail where you have a suspicious condition. If you see pinpoints of bleeding where you scrape off the scale, that is very likely psoriasis. This is called the Auspitz sign, named after its discoverer, a German dermatologist.

The bleeding is due to the fact that the psoriasis scale is attached to the skin, and when you scrape it off, the little plugs that hold it and feed it through fine capillaries are broken causing the tiny red pinpoints. There is really no other skin problem that looks just like this.

Caution: although your skin may be normal, if you have a tendency to psoriasis, and you scratch your skin deeply, you can develop psoriasis in that scratch; though this might take weeks to develop. This is the Koebner phenomenon, where the psoriasis develops in an irritated spot.

If you get an insect bite, psoriasis might develop around the bite. Check the edges of the bite for a dryish condition.

This tendency of psoriasis to develop around any point of irritation, perhaps just in faint traces, provides a possible preview of coming events, which could be triggered in the future by periods of emotional stress, or by physical irritation.

Many people who have psoriasis of the scalp think that they have dandruff. Close examination by you can reveal telltale signs of psoriasis. While dandruff is a general condition of the scalp that usually causes no localized patches, psoriasis is sharply outlined.

A patch is visible. It can be a round patch or an oval patch, or any shape.

When the psoriasis is quite mild or just beginning, it resembles dandruff more closely. Then we call it seborrhiasis—seborrh(ea) + (psor)iasis.

But more typically, psoriasis creates a sharp cutoff between the area of the scalp it is affecting and the adjacent areas of normal scalp.

Some Newer Treatments Now Being Used

Because psoriasis grows like cancer, anti-cancer treatment works on psoriasis.

Methotraxate, which is an antimetabolite used in cancer treatment to stop cells from multiplying, is now being used successfully in the treatment of psoriasis.

Methotraxate should be used only in cases where the psoriatic patient is disabled or incapacitated, and is not responding to usual treatment. In such cases, a stronger therapy is needed, such as this antimetabolite. Methotraxate does have its risks. It can cause a toxic condition, and some people have succumbed to toxemia due to the use of the drug. Liver biopsies, blood tests, and other precautions are advisable before using it.

Methotraxate should not be routine treatment.

The newest treatment for psoriasis at this writing is called PUVA. The P stands for psoralen; the UV for ultra-violet; and the A for the band of ultra-violet light that makes pills work better. The psoriasis patient is given a psoralen pill by mouth. Then, two hours later, he gets into a PUVA light box for a few minutes.

It takes twenty or thirty treatments, but then the psoriasis just melts away, and the skin remains free of it for longer periods.

Again, PUVA is recommended for widespread or total body psoriasis that does not respond to usual treatment. Periodic booster treatments may be needed, because PUVA is still a treatment rather than a cure. In the future, after further research is completed, it may be possible to give PUVA without the light box. The patient might be able to take the pill and just go out into the sun.

One disadvantage of the PUVA treatment is that it could be irritating to the eyes. Special glasses must be worn in the light box, and after treatment for six to eight hours—especially if you live in very sunny areas such as Hawaii or Florida. The psoralen pill is very safe when used under a doctor's direction. But because mice have developed cataracts when exposed to the sun after test treatment, the sunglasses precaution is necessary.

A bonus of PUVA is that you get a good-looking suntan from the treatment. My patients love it.

Sixteen leading medical centers joined together in 1976 to conduct a cooperative clinical study of the promising PUVA program. What triggered this project was a Harvard Medical School report in 1974, by a Department of Dermatology medical team, that twenty-one of twenty-four patients with general psoriasis were able to obtain complete clearing with the treatement.

Other chemicals are currently being tried out in the treatment of psoriasis. These are basically cancer treatment chemicals, which act as poisons to the cancer cells but are relatively safe for healthy cells. When used in psoriasis these chemicals pose the same risks, but a risk taken by a cancer patient may be unwarranted for a psoriasis patient. So what we are trying to do, you might say, is to find safe poisons—poisons that will attack the psoriasis scales, but not the kidneys or other organs.

It takes time to find such a treatment. "Safe" dosages of

arsenic compounds were used to treat skin diseases decades ago, and patients developed skin cancer thirty years later.

If the wheels of progress appear to move slowly, this is because time itself is the vehicle.

Where time is a critical factor—as when a wedding approaches and the bride has psoriasis on her body, or the groom has psoriasis on the penis—a fast acting type of cortisone, injected into the buttocks, remains the best and fastest known treatment today.

Sometimes, when nothing else works, a treatment of coal tar will. This is a black ointment, just like tar. The affected skin is covered with this messy stuff, and then wrapped with a bandage. Coal tar is such a nuisance, staining everything, that this treatment has to be done in the hospital.

A forty-year-old taxi driver who lived alone had watched his psoriasis get worse. Now it was total. He was hospitalized, and covered with this tar. "Feathers, too?" he asked. "No, just this bandage," replied the nurse, as she wrapped his entire body. For twelve days he went through this process, and by then there was enough improvement that he could be released from the hospital. Perhaps one of the newest and most dramatic treatments is the Dead Sea treatment. In Israel, patients with psoriasis go to the Dead Sea, where the water level is lower than sea level, and so the lack of drainage creates a unique salt level that appears to be therapeutic. In addition, this below sea level horizon means more atmosphere to screen out harmful rays of the sun. So the combination of Dead Sea bathing and sun bathing is effective, so effective that physicians all over Europe are sending their psoriatic patients to Israel for treatment.

Final Words to the Psoriatic Patient

Psoriatic patients need patience. Impatience causes stress. Stress contributes to the unwanted condition.

Patience is needed in three ways.

First, patience with the testing of new approaches. Take as an example the new PUVA treatment. The impatience of psoriatic sufferers has resulted in the use of improvised lamps. These "jerry-built" units often do not provide uniform light intensity, require inordinate exposure time, and do not have safety devices.

Many physicians, knowing that side reactions to treatments do not surface immediately, have decided to hold off on PUVA treatments, at least until the present cooperative program has come up with its findings.

Second, while waiting for new, safe, and more effective treatments, psoriatic patients need to be patient with the present treatments. They need to be conscientious in applying medications as directed, day after day, night after night, for whatever time is needed to turn back the psoriasis attack. Psoriatics who become impatient with the treatment and switch to other types of treatment may become patients for other types of dermatitis.

Third, patients need to be patient with life itself. Impatience leads to tension. Any kind of stress feeds the cause of psoriasis. "Cool it." Acquire a philosophical attitude toward life's problems. Don't let other people "get under your skin."

It is easy for somebody else to prescribe patience for you, but I am going to make one final constructive suggestion to help you live with your psoriasis until your present treatment is effective, and until even more effective treatments become available.

When a person gets up from a chair and a shower of scales falls to the floor at his or her feet, the blow to the morale is devastating.

Whatever kind of psoriasis you have, you feel like an outcast—a self-proclaimed leper.

This sense of alienation is the source of great suffering. To alleviate it, psoriatics have been joining together to help each other over their emotional pain. This banding together of psoriatic sufferers is done under the auspices of the National Psoriasis Foundation.*

It all started back in 1966, when Beverly W. Foster of Portland, Oregon, was suffering from psoriasis, and decided that if others who were enduring the same torment as she could get together and communicate, it would be helpful to everybody. Ms. Foster advertised in the personal columns of the newspaper, asking for other sufferers from psoriasis to get in touch with her. The response was overwhelming.

---

*Suite 250, 6415 S. W. Canyon Court, Portland, Oregon 97221

Today, there are such groups meeting throughout the country. They invite dermatologists to speak, and they discuss individual problems. They gain self-understanding, and help boost each other's morale.

One final reminder to the psoriasis-prone—avoid physical and emotional irritation, get moderate amounts of sunlight on your body, follow your physician's instructions, and . . . patience!

The Sun—Skin Enemy Number One

A child cannot live without the sun.

An adult cannot live with the sun.

The sun plays a dual role in our life. A classic among men about women and vice versa is, "You can't live with 'em, and you can't live without 'em." The saying probably applies more accurately to the sun.

A child's body needs the direct rays of the sun to metabolize vitamin D. Even so, only a few minutes a day will suffice. Toxicity can result from excessive amounts of vitamin D. When the bones have fully matured, the need for the direct rays of sunlight is ended.

Life would not exist on earth were it not for the sun. Without sun, our planet would be dark, cold and barren. But there have been millions of people who have grown old before their time, or for whom life no longer exists—because of the sun.

The sun is your skin enemy number one. It ages you, injures you, and eventually can destroy you. In this chapter, I am going to tell you how to retain your youthful look, minimize solar damage to your skin, and survive, forever attractive, on this sunlit planet.

Natural Light Yes— Direct Sunlight No

There is considerable research going on today pointing to the beneficial effects of natural light on animal life, specifically on man. Dr. John N. Ott, in his book *Health and Light,** points out our dependence on the full spectrum of light. Most of us know about photosynthesis, by which plant leaves respond to sunlight to help form carbohydrate. Dr. Ott has uncovered evidence pointing to this same basic principle carrying over into animal life.

Male rats bred in artificial light have to be removed from the female's cage because of irritability and a tendency to cannibalism. But male rats exposed to the full spectrum of natural light are docile, and even help the mother care for the litter.

Experiments with mink breeding indicate that man's baldness may be in large part due to the time he spends under incandescent or fluorescent light and filtered window light.

The latest research is directed at the effect of light on the pineal and pituitary glands, via the retina, and through these glands on the total health of the person.

What these experiments indicate is that light bulb manufacturers may have to go back to their drawing boards in order to produce closer to full-spectrum natural light, and the same for manufacturers of home and auto glass. Indeed, they are already working on this, and on full-spectrum fluorescent lights.

Because full-spectrum fluorescent lights are available, and the full spectrum includes the sunburning, skin cancer causing wave lengths, I tested several different manufacturers' fluorescent bulbs on hairless mice, and found that after one and a half years, all of the fluorescent bulbs tested failed to produce skin cancers in the laboratory animals.

Fluorescent *sun*lamps on the other hand, cause skin cancer in mice. Fluorescent sunlamps provide a high intensity of 290-320 nanometers of ultra-violet light.

The American Cancer Society estimates that some 115,000 new skin cancers are currently being detected each year in the

---

*Devin-Alder Co., Old Greenwich, Conn.; 1974.

United States. Of these, 5,000 will result in death.

What is the primary cause of skin cancer? Over-exposure to the direct rays of the sun.

Anatomy of the Sun

Years ago, man's knowledge of the sun was based on rudimentary astronomy, superstition, and sun-worship.

To the ancient Greeks, the sun was the god Apollo driving his chariot across the sky. To the Egyptians, the sun was the god Ra, sailing his ship across the heavens. The Hopi Indians, the Aztecs of Mexico, the Incas of Peru—and many other peoples—believed themselves to be descendants of the sun or of a sun god.

The "divine right of kings" on which European monarchies were based was said to emanate from the sun; and Japan's emperors were said to be directly descended from the sun.

Today, however, we look at the sun with more scientific eyes. We see it as the nearest of all stars, only 93 million miles away. We know that the sun is some 109 times the diameter of the earth, and some 300,00 times more massive. We know that the heat is so great at the sun's center—20 million degrees centigrade—that atomic nuclei collide with such violence that atoms are transformed from one element to another, and over 500 million tons of hydrogen are transmuted into helium every second!

In this process four million tons of mass are lost by the sun every second. This is the material that is converted into radiant energy, flowing out from the sun's incandescent surface at the rate of one-half million billion billion horsepower per second. Little wonder that the energy crisis has caused scientists to consider the use of solar power.

The earth gets only one half-billionth part of this radiation, but that is enought to keep our planet's temperature comfortably above the absolute zero of outer space. Variations occur as sunspots and magnetic storms rage across the sun's gaseous surface.

When the radiation is analyzed here on earth, scientists use the term "Angstrom" to measure the wave length of the sun's rays—one hundred-millionth of a centimeter.

The present term is "nanometer" with one nm. equal to ten Angstroms. The visible rays are 2,500 to 4,000 Angstroms, and the ultra-violet rays from 2,900 to 3,200 Angstroms are the tanning, burning, and cancer-producing wavelengths.

Now you are familiar with the "business" end of the sun's spectrum. These are the rays that can make you and break you.

What the Sun Can Do for You and to You

The immensity of the sun's power should convince you that its rays penetrate deep into your skin. The tan you seek and receive is only part of the story.

A suntan is the prime motive for most people's attraction to the skin. The bronze look is "in" for Americans. However, it is a curious fact of human nature that, while light-skinned people seek to be tanned, dark-skinned people seek to be less dark.

So people with fair complexions, who can tolerate less sun, go out in it more, and people with dark complexions, who are not as vulnerable to sun damage, tend to stay out of the sun.

If a tan gives you a feeling of attractiveness and improves your self-confidence, then it is important for you to have a tan. A good self-image is a large factor in social and business success.

But: if the way you go about getting that tan also gives your skin a leathery texture, if the sun wrinkles you and makes you look far older than your years, if the periodic suntanning brings on pre-cancerous conditions of the skin, what will happen to your self-image?

"Oh, my skin can take it," a young man said to me. Two years later, I was using liquid nitrogen to freeze and remove two keratoses—pre-cancers of the skin—from his neck.

How much sun can the average skin take? If you mean before there is evidence of deleterious effects, the answer is: none.

That's right. Just a few minutes in the sun can cause marked changes in skin. The skin on your buttocks is the proof—unless you're a nudist. A person's face may show aging signs, but the parts of the body that are never exposed to the sun's rays remain as satiny and smooth as a baby's.

What is more, changes occur beneath the outer layer of the skin which you cannot see, but which are the shadow of future skin events. What we consider to be our skin, that is, the outer layer that burns, tans, or peels, is just the beginning of our skin—the epidermis. The epidermis has many layers of cells, which are constantly being renewed, the dead or dying cells being moved up and cast off throughout the top or outside layer.

Beneath the epidermis is the dermis. This is the "working" part of our skin. Here function the nerves, sweat glands, hair follicles, and blood capillaries. Here is where the real damage can take place.

Thanks to a new method of photography, we can see shadows of problems to come. Not so coincidentally, we use the same ultra-violet rays in this flash picture-taking as cause skin problems.

The left side of the photo below, taken in natural lights, shows a person with no apparent sun damage to the skin. The right side, taken with penetrating ultra-violet light, clearly shows skin problems that are going to surface in the future.

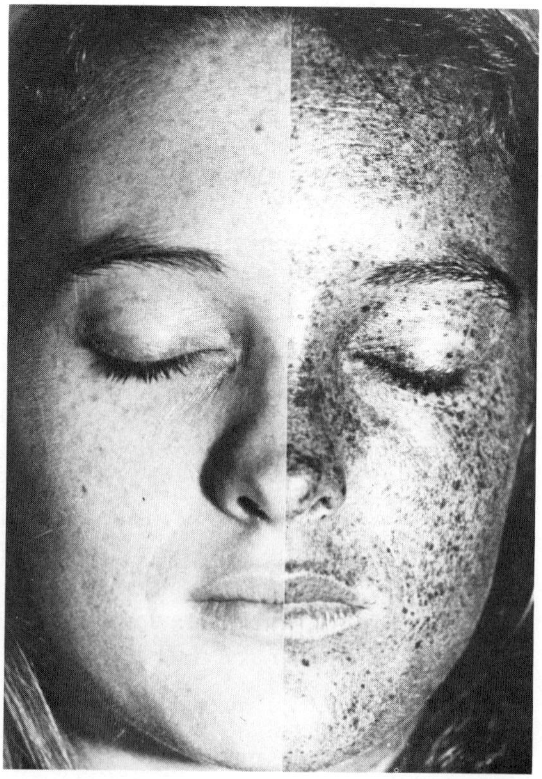

Left side of face: regular photograph shows no problems.

Right side of face: ultra-violet photograph shows sun-caused problems on the way.

How Tolerant of Sun is Your Skin?

You tan. You lose your tan. Does that mean your skin gets a "fresh" start? Unfortunately, no.

The dermis becomes "fatigued." Engineers can estimate how long it takes for metals under vibrational stress (such as aircraft members) to become fatigued. Fatigued metals lose their structural properties. The skin seems to have a limited life-span, too.

This life-span of the skin is directly proportional to the number of hours the skin is exposed to the sun. Some say that the total life of your skin is limited to 100,000 to 200,000 hours of sun exposure. This would mean that the skin of a person sitting three to six hours a day in direct sunlight could live one hundred years. Don't count on it!

Undoubtedly, there have been farmers and fishermen who have survived this kind of exposure. But you and I are likely to get into serious trouble long before we are even half-centenarians.

Some people can survive three hours of midday sun and not get burned. Others turn beet-red in half that time. Just as the epidermis varies in its speed of reaction to the sun among different individuals so the dermis has varying "life spans" measured in total exposure.

We all know that the sun is stronger at midday, stronger on the longest days of the year, and stronger the closer we get to the equator. All three of these factors are due to filtering of the sun's rays by the atmosphere.

At noon on the equator, the sun's rays have only fifty miles of atmosphere to penetrate. This is the shortest vertical route (where the least shadow occurs). As the sun moves away from the vertical and enters the atmosphere at an angle, its rays must go through many more miles of atmosphere, and the rays are weakened accordingly.

Attention skiers; the snow acts as a multi-sided reflector, intensifying the sun's rays from many directions. Also, higher altitudes are like lower latitudes—less atmospheric protection for you.

Obviously, the closer to the equator you reside, the closer to

June 21,* and the closer to noon you expose yourself to sun, the fewer hours you can safely tolerate.

If the sun rays are not weakened, your skin is.

Other important factors are involved. The amount of a pigmentation in your skin is the most important of these. Blond Caucasians can tolerate less sun than brunette Caucasians. The reason is the different pigments of their skins. Pigment is derived from a substance called melanin. Where melanin is produced, darker complexions result. Negroes have a large amount of melanin, albinos none at all. Sun rays cause melanin-producing cells to work overtime. This tanning is a means of protection.

Other metabolic functions are involved in determining sun tolerance level, but no practical measuring devices are available to us.

What *are* available to us are ways and means to have our cake and eat it, too.

Common Mistakes: Sun Protection that is No Protection

"I'll sit in the shade—I'll be okay."

Can't you just see that lobster red skin? Palm trees provide little protection from the tropical sun. Beach umbrellas are just as ineffectual on any United States beaches. The sea and the sand form a giant reflector that bounces searing ultra-violet sun rays at you from all sides, as you sunbathe in false security.

"Cocoa butter—you can't burn with that."

Can't burn? You can be barbecued! Most tanning butters, baby and mineral oils, and lubrication creams and lotions give absolutely no protection to your skin from the ultra-violet rays of the sun.

"I'll put on face coloring (or bronzer). It will block the burning rays."

Bronzing creams block nothing. Their dye is a sun substitute, not a protector. More about this later.

To be effective, products that we apply to our skin must be

*In extreme southern portions of the United States, the noon sun is directly overhead twice—just before and just after June 21.

barriers against the damaging rays of the sun. If they do not actually screen out ultra-violet rays, you are not getting what you are paying for. Lotions, butters, moisturizing oils, bronzes, cosmetic stainers—none of these are sunscreens.

However, there are some products which are indeed ultra-violet ray screens.

How to Recognize Sun Protection

For several years, I have been working on the prevention of skin cancer. We have been losing the fight on skin cancer because we are satisfied to burn off tumors and cut them out, and search out pre-cancerous and cancerous tissue for chemical treatment.

Little has been done in the area of skin cancer prevention. Yet, it's a relatively simple problem. Since 90 percent of skin cancer is sun-related, the target for such prevention research was clear: to find an effective sunscreen, and prove that it reduces or prevents skin cancer.

The sunscreen was easy to find. A chemical has been around a number of years that does protect the skin from ultra-violet rays of the sun. It is included in some commercial preparations. It is called para aminobenzoic acid (PABA). However, since no research had yet been done to determine PABA's cancer-preventive potential, we decided to test it.

We used mice as our "guinea pigs." We exposed the mice to ordinary ultra-violet sun rays, but in order to hasten the process, we also gave them a tumor-producing agent. A control group of nine mice we did not cover with PABA. The control group developed four tumors among them in eight weeks. The PABA groups, divided by age, developed only one tumor among nineteen mice in eight weeks.

So far so good. We continued the experiments twelve more weeks. At the end of that time—twenty weeks in all—the control group of nine mice had developed twenty-eight tumors, while the nineteen PABA-treated mice had only three tumors.

The test continued under different circumstances and under varying conditions. But initial results bode well for PABA—well enough for me to say unequivocally that PABA is an effective sunscreen, and that products containing PABA give the best protection from ultra-violet ray skin damage that we are currently aware of.

Read the labels of the product you buy. Make sure that included in the ingredients is "PABA" or "para-aminobenzoic acid" or "p-aminobenzoic acid." And given the choice between an oil, cream, or alcohol base, choose the alcohol. It penetrates the skin, and gives greater protection.

One such nationally distributed product is Presun. It calls itself a "sunscreen," and it is. This does not mean you do not tan with Presun. It does permit slow, even tanning—safely.

Usually, one application of this type of product provides all the protection you need for the rest of the day, as it resists removal by perspiration. However, if your "day" in the sun is more than two or three hours long, better have a second go at it; and if you take a swim, give yourself another application. PABA works better with time, so you can increase its protection by applying it on areas to be exposed an hour beforehand. If you live in a sunny clime, it is wise to get the PABA habit: apply each morning after washing.

Recently, I conducted a survey of members of a state dermatological society and some thirty pharmacies in that state, to see what sun protection the professonal people were recommending, and what the drugstores were putting on their shelves.

The "top five" sun protectives prescribed, measured in terms of the number of patients advised to use them per month were:

Presun	410
Pabafilm	158
Maxafilm	39
Blockout	20
Solbar	16

It was not surprising to find PABA in a 5 percent alcohol solution heading the list, and the PABA esters and the benzophoenoes following closely, for these are the formulations that zero in on the critical wave length range—2.900–3,200 angstroms: the sunburn spectrum.

How about the pharmacy shelves? Did Presun and Pabafilm get the biggest display space? No, Tanya and Coppertone, the two most widely advertised in that state—and least prescribed by the dermatologists there—were the most lavishly displayed suntan products.

Coconut oil, cocoa butter, and baby oil may be fine on baby's bottom, but despite the message from your TV screen, magazine ads, and taxi and bus advertisements, they afford no protection from sunburn.

You can encourage manufacturers to develop and promote better sun protectives by buying smart yourself and advising your friends and relatives to do likewise.

Some persons are sensitive to PABA, and it can cause irritation to develop. If so, discontinue its use. If the irritation persists, consult your dermatologist. However, most sun-worshippers have reason to rejoice, with PABA around.

"Suntan" without Sun

Men have been using bronzers for years. The more we find out about the sun's cancer-causing rays, the better these bronzers look as the healthier way to get a "healthy" tan.

Bronzers are harmless dyes that give the face a ruddy look. They used to require a moisturizer base, but now they can be applied directly, and they provide a more even tan than the older products.

Bronzers come in squeeze tubes as gels, or in solid stick form. The gels dry faster, but the stick gives better control.

The best way to use a bronzer stick is first, to wash and shave. Do not use an after shave lotion, as the alcohol will make the dye run. Next, take the bronzer and starting at the forehead, work your way down. You can blend dark and light areas by rubbing with the fingertips.

The gel is applied by first rubbing on the palms, then massaging the face. Again, blend with the fingertips or butt of the palm.

The residue on your hands is easily removed with soap and water. The bronzer will not stain collars, and can be removed from the face later by scrubbing with soap and water.

Some men still consider bronzers as makeup. Maybe they are. But if you want that suntanned look, then "make up" the safety that the sun lacks.

What to do about Acute Sun Poisoning

You have no excuse for overdoing sun exposure. Except:

- You met somebody fascinating.
- The surf was up.
- There seemed to be clouds in the sky.
- The boat was becalmed.
- The bridge game went into an extra rubber.
- You couldn't meet anybody fascinating.

"Hi, Bill"
"DON'T TOUCH ME!"
Now what?

You cannot turn a well-done steak into a rare steak. You cannot make your sunburn go away. All you can do is relieve the pain and discomfort. The best treatment for sunburn is cold, wet compresses applied to the skin, also aspirin taken by mouth.

Bland cold creams, ointments, and soothing lotions are the best you can do for your sunburn. Some commercial lotions contain anesthetics that relieve the pain, but these can cause allergic reactions. It would be best to test such lotions out in advance on a small portion of your skin, so that if you later use them on severe sunburn, you will not be adding insult to injury.

Never subject yourself to overdoses of sun—with or without sunscreen.

Be reasonable. Condition your skin. Permit melanin to form—with those protective pigmentations. Here's a guide as to how many minutes to expose yourself to medium to strong sun.

	MINUTES OF EXPOSURE	
	Light Complexions	*Dark Complexions*
First time	15	20
Second time	20	25
Third time	25	30

If you use a sunscreen product, you can double these times. After the third exposure, base your future exposure times on how well you have fared with this schedule.

When you have reached your safe level of tolerance, don't settle for partial shade or an umbrella. Even being dressed and wearing a wide-brimmed hat will not protect your face. All forms of covering help, but there is only one way to totally avoid sun damage—go indoors.

Burning from the sun can be categorized in severity much the same way as burning from fire. First-degree burns via the sun consist of the usual reddening followed by peeling. Second-degree sunburns yield small water blisters. Third-degree burns exhibit more severe blistering and skin eruptions.

This blistering is a sign that lower cells have been damaged or destroyed. The body releases fluids to help protect the inflamed cells in lower layers from direct pressure.

If widespread second-degree burns occur, or if localized third-degree burns occur, see your physician. Burned areas become possible locations for skin cancer to develop, and should be kept under periodic observation.

Skin Cancer: Prevention and Recognition

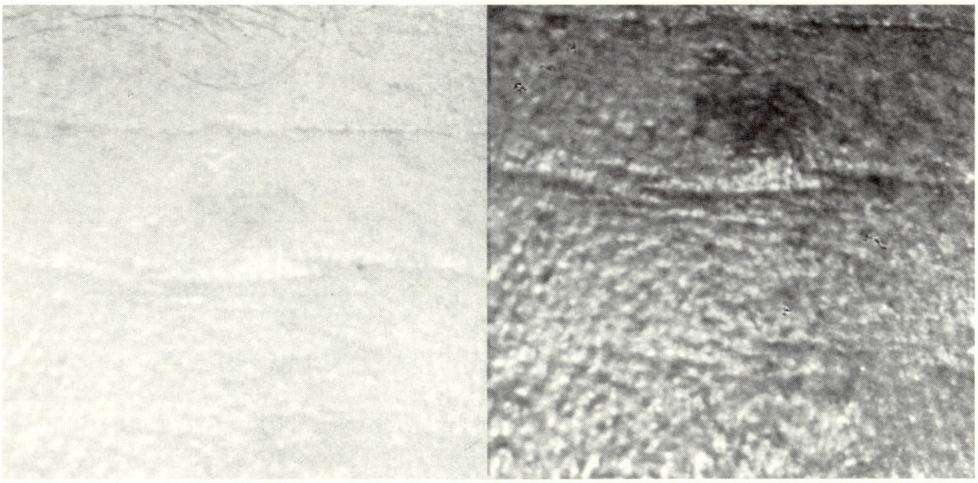

Regular photograph (left) *shows what appears to be an innocent mole on the forehead. Ultra-violet photograph* (right) *permits true diagnosis: cancer.*

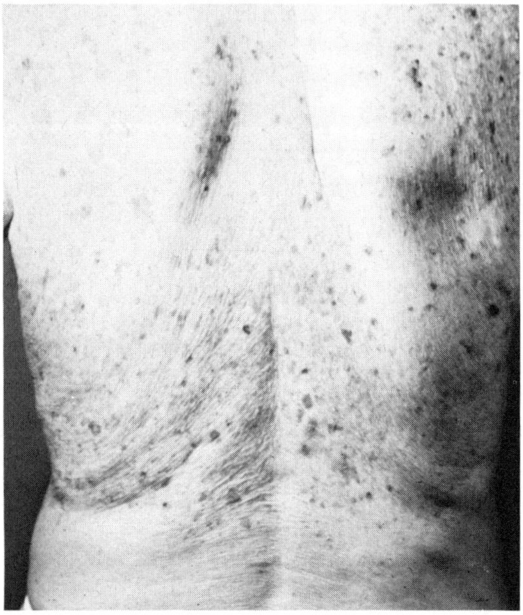

Multiple skin cancers from excessive sun on back and buttocks of seventy-two-year-old man.

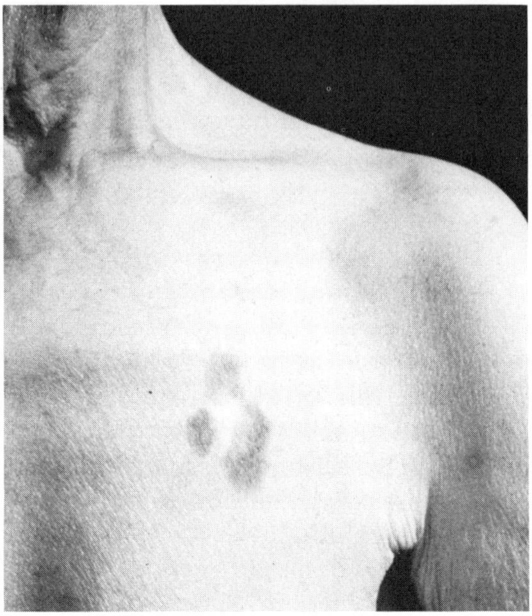

Skin cancer on woman's chest, caused by sun.

Skin cancer, if not recognized and treated, can become as dangerous as other cancers. But fortunately, it is easily recognized and simply treated.

Not all skin cancer is caused by the sun. But 90 percent of the cases reported involve considerable sun exposure.

The sun cannot be blamed for all the difference between the softness of the skin on your buttocks and the skin on your face. Our environment contains irritants other than sun that can lead to skin cancer. Other enemies of your skin are wind, temperature extremes, variations in humidity, dust, and chemical air pollutants.

There are also internal factors that make your skin more sensitive to these irritants. More about these later.

Except for the sun, the skin irritations that can cause cancers are largely man-made. Hot weather that causes us to perspire is harmless. Cold weather that causes us to have to rub away numbness is not a skin irritation. Average weather conditions do not irritate. An exception is frostbite. This is not a common occurrence, but when exposure to extreme cold causes frostbite, extensive skin damage can be produced.

On the other hand, the heat damage caused by man-made saunas or scalding water or steam (if treatments are repeated sufficiently) increases the skin's susceptibility to cancer. And if certain strong chemicals like sulphur compounds and hydrocarbons continue to be introduced into the atmosphere by man, his eyes and lungs will not be the only organs affected. His skin, too, will begin to show destructive effects of these chemicals. Other man-made cancer-causing irritants are coal tar, arsenic compounds, radium and X-rays, paraffin oil, and pitch.

Meanwhile, the prevention of most skin cancer lies in prudent exposure to the sun.

Skin cancer on the bottom lip from pipe smoking.

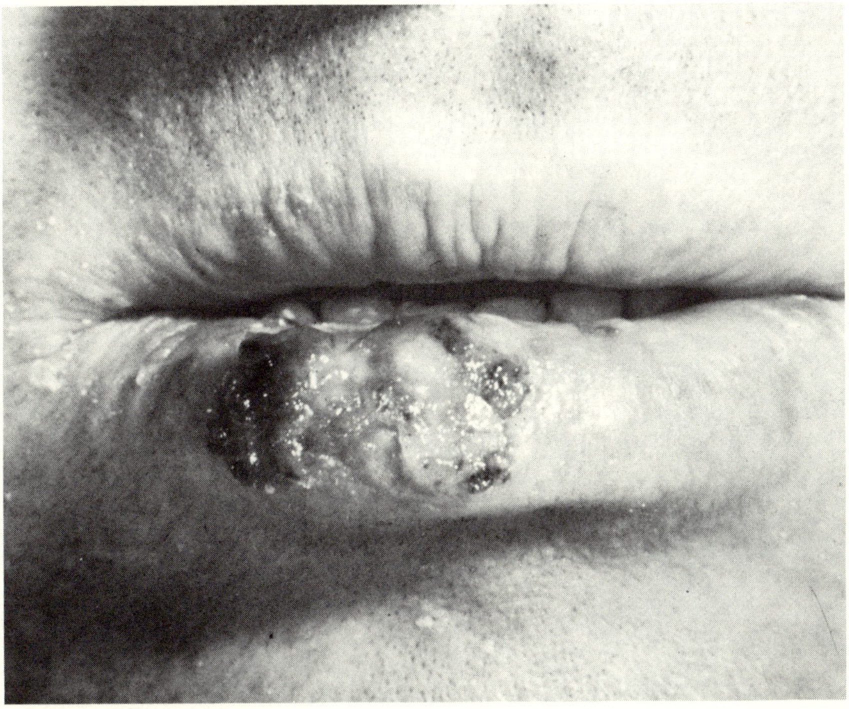

Examine your own skin periodically. Look in the mirror at your face, neck, shoulders, and back. Examine, too, your hands and arms. Have another person help you. Suspect should be any or so-called "liver spot" mole that changes in color and size. Also suspect, and worthy of a visit to your physician, is a sore that does not heal.

Like other forms of cancer, skin cancer consists of abnormal cells that grow uncontrollably. These cells, if not removed, can invade adjacent organisms and may spread to other organs of the body.

Skin cancer can take on many forms. The sore-like form already mentioned is one. Moles are another origin of skin cancer. "Liver spots" are also fertile ground for tumors. So are the acne-like pits that grow deeper or larger, or that bleed. Actually, any brown, reddish, or black nodules or lesions on the skin could be cancerous or pre-cancerous. So could lumps or discolored patches on the lips.

Crater-like skin cancer.

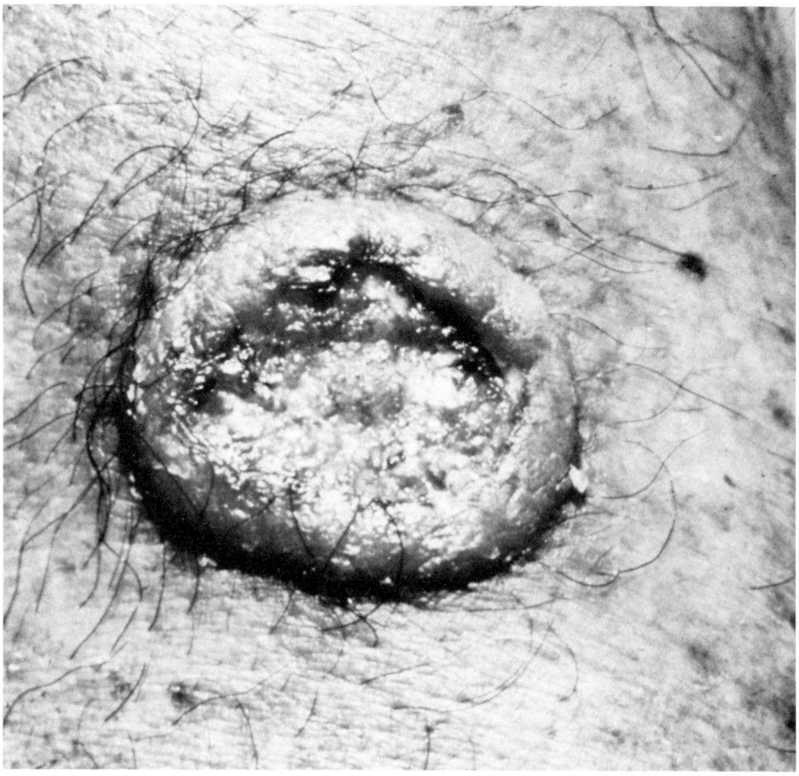

Scaly thickenings on the surface of the skin can be precancerous. These thickenings are called keratoses (singular: keratosis). Keratoses are usually found on the face, neck, chest, and hands, more likely in sun-exposed areas than not.

Some physicians call keratoses "senile spots." However, keratoses have no connection with age or youth. Their connection with amount of sun exposure would seem to me more pertinent.

Not all keratoses become skin cancers. In fact, most keratoses do not. But it is important to spot those that are becoming cancerous in nature. This is done by your doctor taking a small specimen of the keratosis and sending it to the laboratory for a microscopic examination. The pathology report will then guide your physician as to whether or not the keratosis needs to be removed.

Skin Cancer: Treatment

The microscopic testing of skin matter is known as a biopsy. Although skin cancer is frequently recognizable without a biopsy, the process is proper procedure for confirmation, especially if some doubt exists.

There are three general methods of therapy for skin cancer— surgery, chemosurgery, and X-ray. The latter is seldom used today. Sometimes a combination of surgery and chemosurgery is required. One treatment may be all that is needed, or the case may require several treatments.

Sam B. came to my office to have me look at a mole on his shoulder that had become quite large. I examined the mole, and in giving the rest of his upper torso the once over, I spotted an unmistakable pearly nodule.

"You have a skin cancer, Sam," I said, "I'm going to remove it." I held a hand mirror so he could see the cancer. "It appears to be a basal cell cancer, but I'll send some of it to the lab and let you know."

"What does that mean, Doc?"

"It means that once I remove the nodule, you have nothing to worry about. In fact, you may never get another one. Keep your eye open, just in case. If another nodule does show up, then it increases the odds that additional nodules will follow. That means less sun for you."

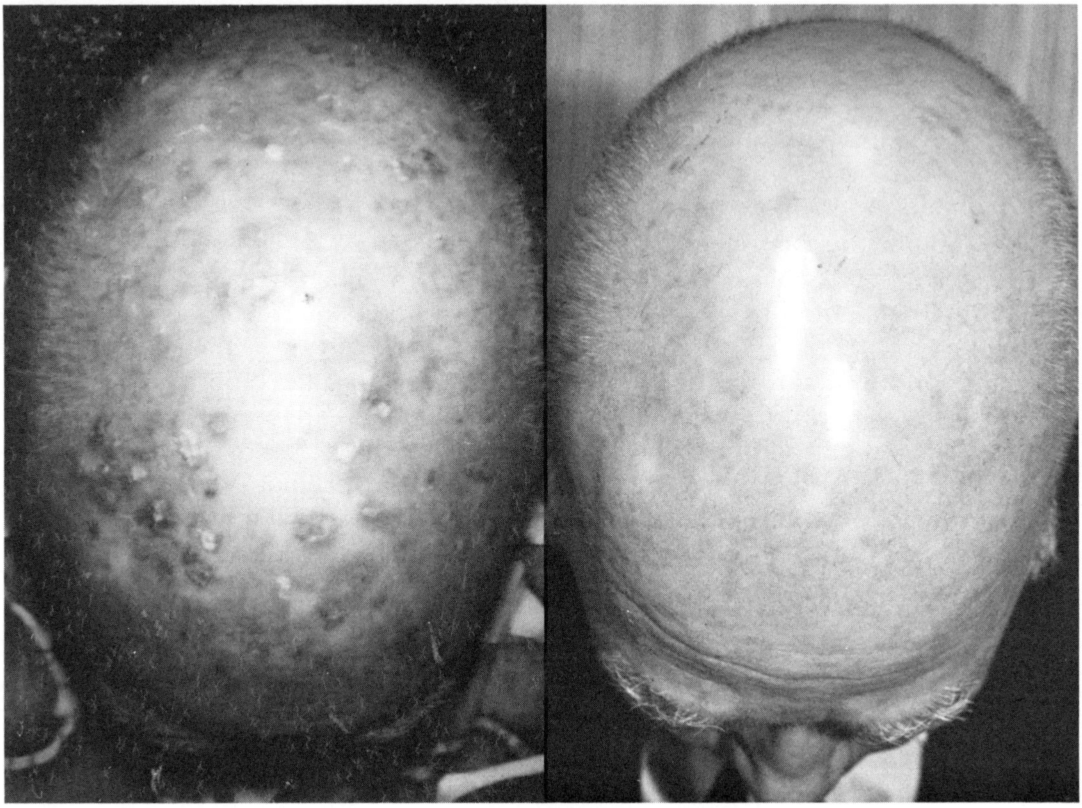

Multiple skin cancers on scalp before (left) *and after* (right) *treatment with anti-cancer cream.*

We chatted about pros and cons of the sun as I readied a cryospray.

"I am going to freeze this off, Sam. You may feel a tingling, burning, or cold sensation for a few minutes, as I spray on this liquid nitrogen."

In a few minutes, the job was done. I froze the enlarged mole, too.

"It will take a few days to a week, possibly more, for these to drop off. I'll call you when the biopsy report is in. I will also call you for a yearly checkup, just as your dentist might."

"Thanks, Doc. Glad that mole caused me to come in."

Had Sam been observant, he could have saved himself a peck of trouble. It is a year now, and he has shown no further sign of skin cancer.

Freezing therapy is rapidly becoming the most widely-used method of removing cancers and pre-cancers. Cryosurgery is also effective for moles, warts, and acne. It is a relatively painless, and properly applied, does a clean job of removal. I prefer a spray, but a freezing preparation can also be applied with a cotton- tipped applicator from a thermal jar.

After freezing, the skin may turn red in that spot, then dry, and peel.

You may wash, shower, swim, or use cosmetics while this is taking place. You may even go out in the sun. If you get a great deal of sun exposure, the frozen site may temporarily turn a shade or two darker than the surrounding skin.

Yes, the common types of skin cancer are easy to get rid of, but remember—skin cancer is even easier to get.

Light Sensitive Skin

All sun safety rules go down the drain occasionally for some people. Severe burning occurs with relatively short exposure time. Burning can be general, or localized in one spot.

Sunburn is due to a temporary condition known as photosensitivity. Photosensitivity seems to be due to certain substances that are found in food, cosmetics, and medications. These substances can cut down your tolerance of the sun by 90 percent.

Some people have this condition permanently. They are allergic to the sun. This is due to a metabolic condition, and seems to be more prevalent among those with extremely light complexions. These people become adjusted in their life-style to get along with this condition.

People with tattoos can be extremely photosensitive. Often, years after tattooing, the tattoos cause adjacent skin problems due to the photosensitivity of the dyes used. Other than skin grafting or dermabrasion, the choice for sufferers from tattoo-caused skin complaints is to avoid the sun.

However, the rest of us, troubled only with occasional photosensitivity, can learn to identify the substances that cause the condition, then eliminate these substances; or, if this is not possible, then to avoid the sun when we are using photosensitive substances.

Photosensitivity can be manifested not only as sunburn, but also as blemishes, eruptions, and rashes.

If you want to be a sleuth and track down the cause of your aggravated reaction to the sun, here are some clues:

COMMON PHOTOSENSITIZERS		
Foods	*Lotions, Dyes, Cosmetics*	*Medicines*
Parsnips	Most antibacterial soaps (Zest, Dial, Safeguard, Phase III, Lifebuoy)	Thorazine
Celery	Many blue dyes (Aniline, Trypan, etc.)	Sulfonamides
Figs	Bithional	Tetracycline*
Many greens	Perfumes containing oil of Bergamot (Jade East, Shalimar)	Iodine
Oil of vanilla		Bromine
Oil of lime		Some antihistamines
Cyclamates		Some barbiturates
		Nalidixic acid
		Quinine

* Demethylchlorotetracycline

The Sun's Secret Weapon

This chapter will not make me popular with sun- worshippers. They will probably remind me that an outdoor life, close to nature, is a healthy life. They may even quote Emerson: "There is no object so foul that intense light will not make it beautiful."

To which I would respond with a quotation from James Thurber: "There are two kinds of light—the glow that illumines, and the glare that obscures."

The glare of the bronzing sun is obscuring to millions of people lolling on beaches, rooftops, and backyards an inescapable truth: The sun is aging your skin, sapping its vitality, drying, cracking, and wrinkling it.

Are you willing to trade one day now as a tanned Venus or Adonis for three days in not-so-later life as a wrinkled prune?

Your skin seems to remember. It is like a computer that totals all the photons received from the day you were born. Then it comes up with the readout—on your face and neck.

It does not matter how many facials you give yourself, how much yoga you do, what vitamins you take. So many photons add up to so many wrinkles.

Go ahead. Moisturize, cream, pat, powder, mudpack, lift, steam, sauna-bake, exercise, massage. At least that will keep you out of the sun.

Here is the anatomy of that old, wrinkled look. The dermis, or main understructure of the skin, is composed of several fibrous tissues, some hard, and some soft. From birth to maturity, these fibers change from a preponderance of soft tissues to a preponderance of hard tissues, giving us a firm, youthful look.

Enter the sun. Its ultra-violet rays attack the dermis; hard fibers lose resilience and turn soft. The skin sags.

Wouldn't it be nice if sagging skin gave us more dimples? It doesn't: it spells wrinkles.

Sagging skin also spells "liver spots," dryness, and the precancerous and cancerous skin tumors we have already discussed, not to speak of comparable problems with the hair and nails.

Maybe some day, we will invent products that restore youth to skin. Meanwhile, the epidermis stands guard, keeping out enemies (except ultra-violet rays) and friends alike. So, were a "fountain of youth" discovered, medical science would still have to find a way to get it past the epidermis into the sagging tissues of the dermis.

Still think how lucky you are. Can you keep your heart forever young? Your liver? Your lungs? You *can* keep your skin forever young. The proof is your buttocks. Contemplate them.

And use a sunscreen—or stay out of the sun!

Blemishes, Warts, Allergies

Remember Mark Twain's Tom Sawyer telling Huckleberry Finn how to get rid of warts? You go into the woods at midnight, back up against a spunk-water stump and command: "Barleycorn, Barleycorn, Injun-meal shorts, spunk-water, spunk-water, swaller these warts." Well, I have news for you. It works.

And so do smallpox inoculations for warts; hot water baths for warts; vitamin B-complex for warts; and scores of other treatments for warts, including hypnosis and psychotherapy. In the latter, perhaps, lies the clue. There is a theory that people have neutralizing antibodies in their blood once they get the wart virus. These various therapies, including hypnosis and Tom Sawyer's magic words, are thought to activate the immunizing process of these antibodies, through expectation and belief. Still a theory, but it serves to explain some of the fascinating aspects of the coming and going of warts.

In this chapter, we will also be fascinated by the skin's ability to cry out against certain substances, and the detective work we need to do to identify these "allergies."

Fighting the War Against Warts

Warts are the most common tumors that doctors see. A

tumor is a lump or a growth. Warts are skin tumors. The word "tumor" often pushes a panic button, as people identify tumors with cancer. Very few tumors are or become cancerous, especially when you consider that warts are tumors, and warts are not cancers. Warts are the home of a virus. They are a benign lesion, and they rarely become cancerous.

The wart virus likes to make its home on the skin, but it also likes mucous membranes such as the mouth, or the opening of the vagina, anus, and penis. In fact, warts grow more rapidly on these areas because they are warm and moist, conditions in which the virus thrives.

The virus can spread to other parts of the body if the wart is picked, scratched, or touched.

Contrary to popular opinion, warts do not come from touching toads. Toads and frogs may have their own viruses, but those viruses are viruses that thrive in amphibians. Children do not get a wart virus from a frog; they get a wart virus from other children.

Warts are all from the same virus, but they can look quite dissimilar. A wart on the finger can look very different from a wart on the anus. This is due to the difference in locale, not in the virus. A house built of logs in timber country looks quite different from a house built of bricks in clay country. A finger or hand wart might be a "digitate wart," which projects away from the skin like a tiny finger, whereas a wart in the anus might look like a coral formation. Other wart locations might yield "trees," "flowers," or "bushes."

Warts grow slowly, and stay with you quite awhile. Warts may bleed if scraped or shaved, because they contain a blood supply. Sometimes you may think you have gotten rid of the "seed" of the wart. What may look like a seed is really just a spot of coagulated blood.

A plantar wart grows on the bottom of the foot. It is called a "plantar wart" not because it is produced by a different virus, but because "plantar" is the anatomical name for that area of the body. Similarly, a wart on the palm of the hand is called a "palmer wart."

Some warts are a minor venereal disease. They can be spread by sexual intercourse. I say "minor" because venereal warts do not usually create any secondary problems, and may disappear spontaneously.

Leave a wart alone, and it may go away in one or two years. This is the life story of most warts. But a wart on the tip of the nose, or some other cosmetically or socially embarrassing location should be treated and not left to the time cure.

You can treat warts effectively at home. Every one of your friends and neighbors can tell you how, including devotees of Mark Twain. But there are some proven, effective medical treatments.

One proprietary (over-the-counter) preparation is Compound W; it includes an acid that eats away the wart. You can also buy a 40 percent salicylic acid plaster. I often prescribe this. First, you soak the affected part of the body in hot water, or take a bath. Then you take a single-edge razor blade and slice the

Plantar warts.

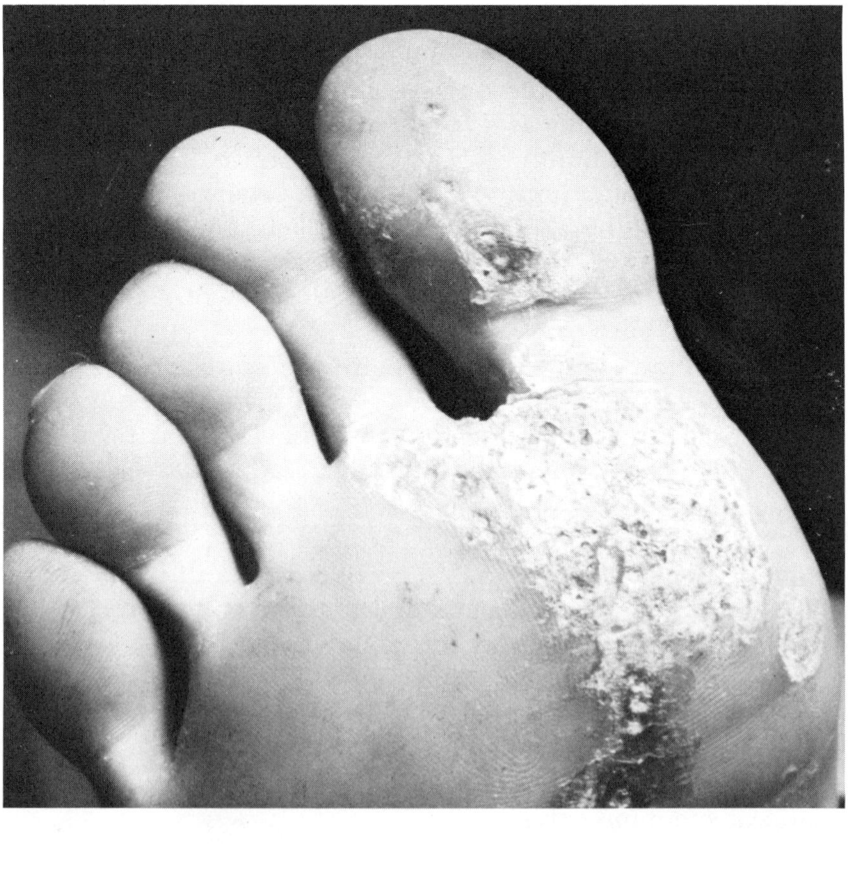

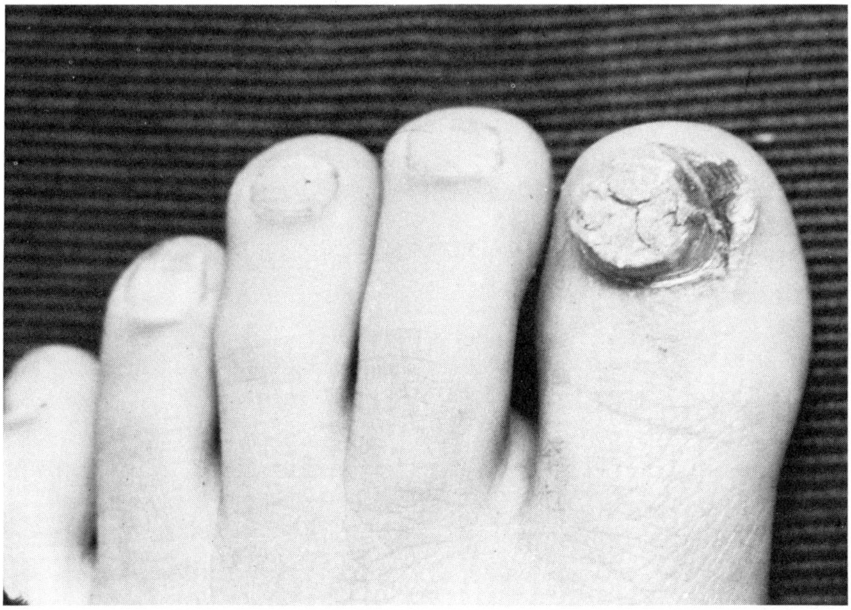

Warts on big toe.

wart down even with the skin, and scrape away any mushy interior matter. Do *not* use your fingernail. Dry the skin, and put on the salicylic acid plaster. Use a piece large enough to just cover the wart. Try not to put the plaster on the surrounding tissue. Keep the plaster in place with a band-aid or adhesive tape. Leave it on for one or two days, and then repeat by starting again with the bath.

Do not use a plaster on tender areas like the penis skin or mucous areas, as it can be irritating. The same applies to Compound W.

Sometimes the use of formaldehyde is effective for warts; this substance is also sold over the counter. Formaldehyde is a pickling solution, used to preserve tissue. Formaldehyde works by drying the skin. As the skin dries, the wart subsides.

Another group of medicines that work for warts are acne medicines. These also dry the skin. (See the second chapter of this book.)

If the skin gets too dry, do not lubricate as with Vaseline. Just stop treating the wart for a few days, then start again. Also, do not keep warts covered when using these preparations. Covering warts tends to increase the temperature and humidity, which the virus loves, so it makes plans to expand its home instead of to move out.

Of course, if a child's wart is being treated and the child tends to scratch at it, the lesser of the two evils is to keep the wart covered.

If the wart does not go away when you treat it, then see your doctor.

How Your Doctor Treats Warts

The electric needle seems to be the first thing that a doctor thinks of when faced with the removal of a wart.

However, I do not feel that the electric needle is necessarily the best way to remove warts, and many of my colleagues agree. The electric needle usually leaves a scar. We do not like to create scars unless there is a compelling reason to do so. A wart is not cancer, nor is it threatening in any way.

If we have to use the electric needle to burn off the wart (which leaves a small scar), we do; but there are alternatives that are well above the needle on the list of preferred treatments.

I would prefer to treat warts with the formaldehyde and acne-treating preparations that I mentioned for home use before resorting to the electric needle. I would also prefer to use cryosurgery, freezing off the wart with liquid nitrogen.

This freezing process is my favorite, and also the patient's favorite. I like cryosurgery because it gives the best results. The patients like it because there is no injection, no mess, and no interruption of their activities.

Occasionally, warts have to be removed by surgery. We prefer not to cut out warts, because they can grow on the incision line and double the trouble.

One well-known dermatologist in Hawaii treats warts with aloe. The syrupy liquid from the leaves of this house plant is soothing to the skin, and valuable for many skin problems, But I think this dermatologist would agree that the therapeutic value of aloe's use for warts is largely "suggestion."

But never underestimate the power of suggestion!

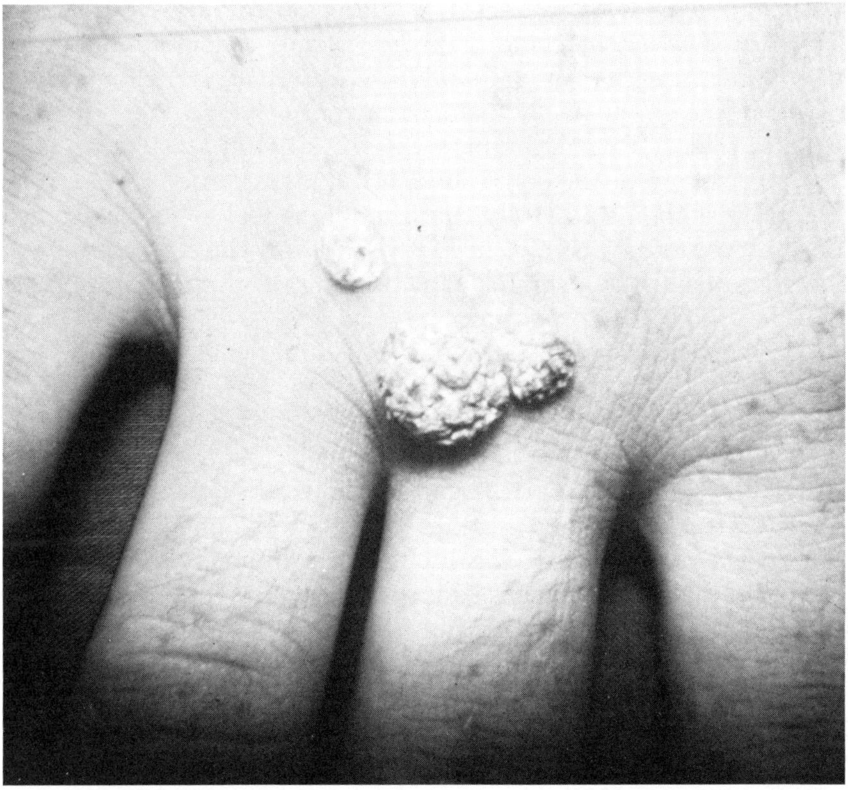

Warts on back of hand.

Why Hypnosis Works for Warts

Holly is nine years old, and in the fourth grade. She has warts on both hands and on her face. The warts started when Holly was in first grade and gradually spread, increasing at a faster rate in the last twelve months. Holly now has thirty-one warts. She is teased in school, where she is called "warty face." Her grades have gone down. Various preparations have not worked. Holly's mother has now accompanied her to a clinic where hypnotherapy will be tried.

The hypnologist asks Holly which side of her body she would like him to work on first. She chooses the left side—her left hand and the left side of her face.

"When I lower my hand, I want you to close your eyes." The doctor lowers his hand. Holly cooperates and closes her eyes.

"Now imagine you are walking carefully down a long flight of stairs as I count backward from twenty-five to one. Twenty-five . . . twenty-four . . . twenty-three . . . twenty-two . . . ."

At the end of the countdown, Holly was quite relaxed. The hypnologist then told Holly that she might feel a tingling sensation in the warty areas of her left hand and the left side of the face, and that when she felt that tingling, it was a sign that the warts would begin to disappear.

"It might take a week or possibly longer. But they will soon be gone."

When the session was over, Holly said it was fun, and rushed out to tell her mother.

Holly's left side warts began to shrink after the first session. Shortly after the second session, a wart over her left eyelid fell off. At the third session, so much improvement was evident on the left side, that Holly agreed it was time to begin the right side. It responded, too. By the end of the fifth session, Holly had lost twenty-six warts. Her face was clear. She had two small warts on her left hand and three on her right. Her classmates no longer teased her, and she was once again getting "A" marks.

This was an actual case reported in the *American Journal of Clinical Hypnosis** by members of the Department of Psychiatry and Dermatology at the Massachusetts General Hospital in Boston.

Nobody can fully explain what happens, when through hypnotism, the subconscious mind is instructed to make changes in the body and then the changes occur.

Certainly, it is our mind that operates our body. It is the stress, anxiety, and tension that our mind experiences that can interefere with the perfect operation of the body.

When you relax and see your problems lessening and your blessings increasing, you are giving yourself a "tonic." That tonic can relieve ulcers, high blood pressure, and a myriad of other ailments—including skin problems like warts.

Emotions affect the blood supply to the skin. Emotions af-

---

*July, 1972, by Owen S. Surman, M.D., C.M., Sheldon K. Gottlieb, M.D., and Thomas P. Hackett, M.D.

fect gland secretions. Emotions affect levels of resistance to germs—and emotions affect the wart virus.

Knowing this, one young man went to a counselor with his warts. They were on his anus. He did not want the pain of treatment there. He was asked what in his life was "bugging" him. He told of his relationship with his girlfriend, which was not going well. They had decided to split. He took her to the airport. When he returned home, she was waiting for him. She had changed her mind. This happened repeatedly. "How many times?" he was asked. "Nine." "And how many warts do you have?" "Nine."

The numerical correlation is probably coincidental. But the physiological location being analogous to the "exiting" aspect of the problem is probably not coincidental. Psychologists and psychiatrists are finding many such correlations between the location of a symptom and its emotional cause.

P.S.: The young man finally solved his exiting girlfriend problem (she boarded and remained on the plane), and the anus warts disappeared.

Hypnotism does not provide a direct treatment of the wart. But when the psyche is calmed down and assurance replaces anxiety, the body responds in its natural way. This may have something to do with the blood supply, or with the immunization process.

You can use the aloe plant, or purple water, or a magic incantation to cure warts. If a person is suggestible—that is, has confidence in the procedure—it may work. Children are more suggestible than adults; so the "magic" incantation worked well for Huckleberry Finn.

When I was in the army, at Ford Gordon in Augusta, Georgia, I treated a number of fascinating cases of warts. One of these was a man with large warts on the index finger of his right hand. The warts were so big that he could not insert his finger into the trigger mechanism of a rifle. He was discharged. Was that his body's way of responding to his "I want out" emotions?

The Future for Warts

Another man at Fort Gordon had warts that completely covered the soles of both feet. He was a picker—he kept picking at the warts when they first appeared, and they spread rapidly. Also, he was an emotionally unstable person, and this did not help his immunization mechanism any. He got warts on his fingertips, too, where they spread after he picked the warts on his feet. He could not put his boots on.

Because this man had been in the service so long, it was too complicated a procedure to give him a medical discharge; so we treated him. We put him in the hospital, and we cut and scraped and pared and froze, and finally, after four or five months, we got rid of all of those warts.

We got to know more about warts from that one case than from perhaps a score of others. We could see the way the wart virus acts, how it spreads, and how it can be inhibited.

Warts are infectious. They are the third most common skin disease treated by dermatologists. I am convinced that just as we have stopped the polio virus, we will one day bring the wart virus to its terminus. We have also eradicated smallpox from the world. Whether we conquer warts by a vaccine or a pill, conquer it we will.

Allergies—the Things Your Skin Dislikes

Some noses dislike pollen—result: hayfever. Some stomachs dislike lobster—result: stomach distress. Some skins dislike wool—result: a rash.

These "dislikes" cause allergic reactions. "Dislike" is not a very scientific word.

Would you prefer this? At the first exposure to a foreign substance, plasma cells form special antibodies for protection against that substance. These antibodies, which have been released into the blood stream, may become attached to cells in the tissues, such as skin cells. If the same foreign substance enters the body again, it can react with these antibodies in the skin cells. Disturbances then occur, and the cells disrupt.

This is the start of an allergic reaction.

Dermatologists treat allergies constantly; they are a major problem. Some allergies are due to substances taken internally, such as foods, medicines, or inhalants. Other allergies are due to external substances that come into physical contact with the body. These substances can come from pets, cosmetics, clothing or myriad other sources, and therein lies the complexity of the problem.

The allergist usually takes care of allergies resulting from substances taken internally. The dermatologist ususally takes care of the external contact allergies.

Both types of allergies can appear on the skin. Both types of allergies can have internal effects.

The most common allergies treated by the allergist are hayfever, rose fever, and food-related reactions. To identify the cause, allergists do scratch testing. They put a chemical or substance on the skin. When the skin forms a bump, it is a sign that the person is allergic to that chemical or substance.

In contrast to the allergist's scratch testing, dermatologists do patch testing. This consists of putting samples of suspected substances under little patches of adhesive, usually on the back, to see which substance might cause a reaction.

Eczema is a general term meaning a rash-like condition of the skin. Contact dermatitis is eczema. So contact allergies in effect cause eczema.

Itching is the main problem caused by allergies. People could live with most kinds of eczema, if it were not for the itching.

We dermatologists need to take our patients' itching seriously. Itching not only invites but almost commands scratching. And scratching almost invariably causes secondary infection. This can mean blood poisoning.

You put on a new watch. After a few days, you notice a red patch on your wrist under the metal of the watch. You do not need patch tests to identify the culprit. You know it is the watch. You do not go to a doctor for a medicine to enable you to wear the watch without an allergic reaction. He probably could not help you. You merely take off the watch.

But, you say, the watch was a gift. You want to wear it. The donor would be hurt if you chose not to wear it. Then wear it, say I, but put some scotch tape or clear nail polish on the back of the watch, so that the metal does not touch your skin.

More likely, you will not know why your skin is itching and red. You may think it is due to some cosmetic, as did the secretary I told you about in a previous chapter, who experienced no relief when she stopped using her mascara. Good reason. It was not the mascara that was irritating her eyes, but the photocopy chemical which she was touching, and transferring to her eyes when she rubbed them.

The basic treatment for a skin allergy is to identify the irritating substance and discontinue contact with that substance.

Meanwhile, though, we do want to relieve the itching, and the swelling, if present.

The best treatment for both itching and swelling is cold packs. Also, the use of antihistamine or cortisone is effective to reduce serious itching.

The process of identifying the cause of an allergic reaction is a bit like Sherlock Holmes's sleuthing. The dermatologist needs to go into a detailed history of past illnesses or allergic reactions, and he needs to get an in-depth account of the patient's activities both at home and at work.

The dermatologist then has available to him a number of substances that duplicate "families" of common allergy-causing substances.

A series of band-aids, each containing a different suspected substance, is placed on the upper back. The location of the allergy does not matter. These band-aid patches are still placed on the back. The reason is that the back is a large, unseen-by-the-public "laboratory," and the allergy will occur on the skin here, just as it did on the skin elsewhere.

There may be twenty or thirty of these patches, each with multiple chemicals in the creams they contain. The patches are kept on the skin for two days. At the end of that time, the patient returns, and the skin under the patches is examined. Wherever there is redness or blistering, the substances or chemicals on the patches are products to whch the patient is allergic.

Let's say that one patch contains a number of chemicals associated with rubber and its manufacture. The patient should then be able to identify the rubber product, contact with which is causing the problem. If the patient works in the rubber industry, additional tests might have to be conducted in order to narrow the finger of guilt to a specific chemical.

There is no immunization procedure for allergies. The patient must use his newly-acquired information to avoid contact with the cause of the allergy. The rubber worker would have to protect or adjust. The office worker who was rubbing her eyes after photocopying might have to wear protective gloves—and stop rubbing.

Urushiols—Ubiquitous and Poisonous

Poison ivy, oak, and sumach all cause contact dermatitis. We will cover treatment of these pesky rashes in the following chapter. I would like to say now that some of these substances can stay active for thousands of years. You can buy an antique from the Orient, and get a poison ivy rash because the Japanese lacquer on the antique—the sap of the lacquer tree—is still "alive."

One of my patients was a thirty-five-year-old traveling salesman. He had contact dermatitis, and his history went something like this: As a youngster living on a Pennsylvania farm, he developed eruptions on his hands after milking cows. As a teenager, he developed rashes on his knees and forearms after "playing in the grass." As an adult, he developed blisters on his hands after playing golf in Georgia, and after changing a tire in California. He developed a ring on his buttocks while traveling. More recently, he had bought a Mah-Jongg set, and suffered rashes. A new shirt gave him a rash after he wore it for the second time.

Now he had come to Hawaii to "escape." After sitting at a bar, he got a rash on his elbows. Now there was a rash on his hands—why, he did not know.

I did not have to use patch tests for this case. The clues were loud and clear.

Poison ivy was transferred from the Pennsylvania meadow to the udder of the milked cow. "Playing in the grass" provided another contact with the ivy. Poison sumac in the rough of the Georgia golf course and poison oak along the California highway did their job. The ring on the patient's buttocks was from a lacquered toilet seat. There was a lacquer finish on the Mah-Jongg case, and also on the bar he had leaned on. The laundry mark on the shirt irritated his neck. All these substances were of the same general poison family we will call "urushiol," from the Japanese, meaning the sap from the lacquer tree.

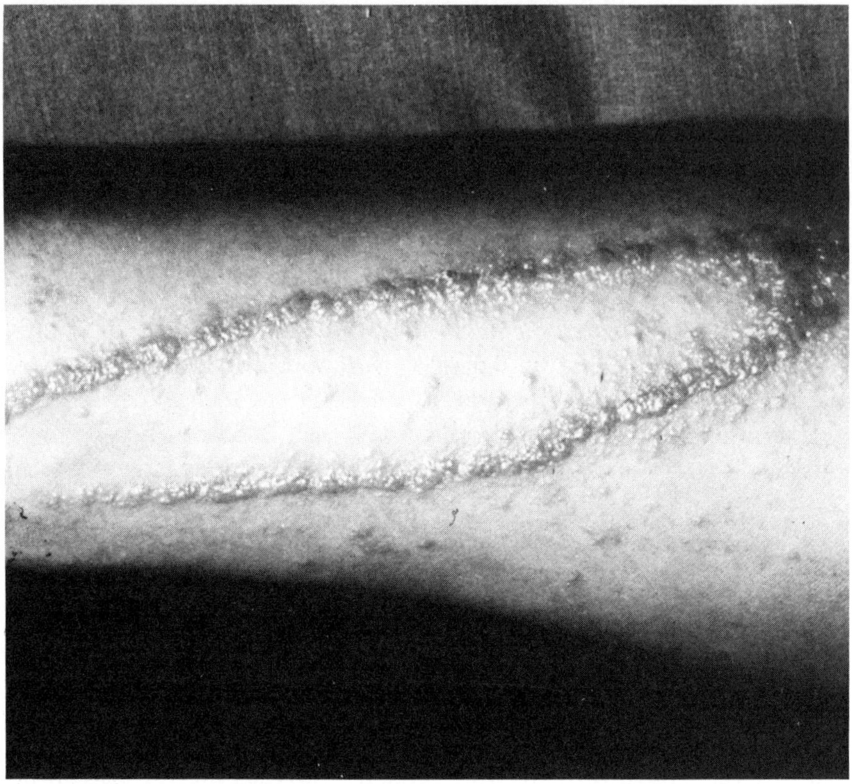

Mango dermatitis on arm of allergic man.

What about his hands? In Hawaii, the most common source of the urushiol-type poison is the king of fruits—the mango. "While here, have you had any contact with mango?" I asked.

"I sure have," he replied. "Picked and ate them day before yesterday."

People who are alllergic to urushiol-type substances are reacting to a chemical found in these substances, all of which belong to a family of trees called anacardiacea. Urushiol, as troublesome a word to mouth, is still easier to pronounce than that. So I frequently make references to the "ubiquitous urushiols."

In the following chapter we will identify the ubiquitous urushiols more specifically, and spell out ways to alleviate the discomfort they can cause.

Clothing Allergies—Shoe to Hat

In New York, a patient came to me with swollen feet. She was a middle-aged housewife. She had bought a new pair of shoes. The shoes fit fine, and were very comfortable, but now she could not wear them (or any other shoes); her feet were that swollen. Her feet were also itching, and the itching areas were oozing with a fluid.

The clues immediately pointed to the new pair of shoes as the culprit. And so it was. The shoes had a black dye. The sweat from the woman's feet leached the black dye from the shoe onto her skin. Wherever the black dye appeared to be less on the shoe, there she had the rash and oozing on the corresponding areas of her feet. I gave her the patch test to confirm her allergy to the dye.

The treatment was not confined to getting this woman a refund on the shoes. She was given an injection of cortisone to relieve the itch, and told to stay off her feet. Being in a horizontal position caused less accumulation of body fluids in her feet, and the swelling soon subsided. Explaining that the black dye in the shoe was paraphenylenediamine, I warned her to avoid clothing that might have this black dye, and also never to dye those gray hairs on her head with a black dye, or she could have the same allergic reaction on her scalp.

Clothing can also be a source of allergic reactions. Wool clothing is "poison" to some people, cotton is poison to others. Certain synthetic fibers cause allergic reactions in some people. Or the dyes in the fabric can be the culprits.

The band of a hat, the chain of a necklace, the leather of a purse—all should be regarded as possible causes of a skin allergy.

If you are suspicious that a watchband is causing an irritation on your wrist, put the watch on your other wrist, and see if the irritation moves over there.

Be a detective.

Contact dermatitis can be recognized and identified from other types of rashes because it follows sharp outlines—where the substance touches the skin. Also, contact dermatitis usually itches more than other types. In fact, it usually begins as just an itch.

The itch may be followed by redness. Then small blisters may form. Giant blisters may take the place of the small blisters, as the small blisters join together.

When the dermatitis spreads, it is not because you touched the blisters and then touched another place on your skin. It spreads because you touched the poisonous substance or substance to which you were allergic, and spread the rash that way. Sometimes the allergy takes a couple of days to show up in a second place.

There is a substance that you can buy over the counter called silicone cream. Put silicone cream on the skin, and you may protect the skin in that area from being irritated by a substance to which you are allergic—like the wristwatch.

Eventually, the skin will develop its own protection to the irritating substance. The skin will literally get hardened to it.

What to do About Hives

Hives are allergic reactions to substances taken internally.

There are exceptions. Some people get hives from ice. These people get hives where the ice touches their skin. Some people get hives from the sun.

Hives are generally related to ingested foods or beverages, or to something inhaled, or to a medicine injected.

Hives are itching blotches, usually elevated. The color of the blotches ranges from white to red. Hives may disappear in a few hours, reappearing later in the same or other places.

Penicillin is a common cause of hives. People who know that they are allergic to penicillin will tell their doctor. However, what many people don't know is that penicillin is not only found in a hypodermic needle. It is also in Roquefort cheese and bleu cheese. Penicillin can be in meat when the animal was given penicillin for some problem. You eat the hamburger, and wonder why you got hives. A cow can have an infection of the udder. Penicillin is used: it gets into the milk; you get hives.

Penicillin is also found in pills and ointments. The drug really should not be used this way. These latent sources of penicillin can evade the most expert Sherlock Holmes. Lists of the sources of penicillin are available; ask your doctor.

Aspirin causes hives, too. The hives go away in a day or so, when the aspirin has left the system. The patient may then brush his teeth with a mentholated toothpaste. Back come the hives!

Menthol, or methyl salicilate, is related chemically to the salicylic acid of aspirin. Mentholated smoke will do the same, whether you inhale your own cigarette or the smoke from someone else's cigarette.

The treatment for hives is an antihistamine preparation, obtainable only by prescription.

You can help yourself at home by taking an over-the-counter cold preparation, many of which—like Contac— contain a low dosage of anti-histamine. But some of these preparations also include aspirin, so inquire at your pharmacy or read the fine print on the package. Ask your pharmacist about some weak antihistamine preparations that he should have in stock.

Penicillin and aspirin are the most common causes of hives. If I had to name a third cause of hives, it would be seafood.

You don't have to be a Sherlock Holmes to track this one down. If you eat shrimp and get hives, and you eat shrimp again and get hives, you get the message.

Sometimes, you get hives from shrimp once, but never again. It is likely that the shrimp ate something to which you are allergic.

You can get hives from strawberries, chocolate, and many other foods.

Use cold compresses on hives. If the hives persist, or get worse, see your doctor. Hives can spread outside as well as inside the body. Inside the body they can cause dizziness, breathing difficulty, and even death.

If you wheeze or have any other symptoms, call your doctor; he will probably have you meet him at the hospital.

If hives persist for weeks, have them investigated. Hives can be an external manifestation of an internal condition.

Hives that last a couple of weeks or even longer are not necessarily cause for that call to the doctor, providing you can function satisfactorily at home and at work.

Eczema—Atopic Allergy

Another kind of allergy is called "atopic." Atopic allergy, atopic dermatitis, atopic eczema—these are all synonyms.

People with asthma, hayfever, and eczema have genetic

disturbances. They are more sensitive in certain ways, and so develop an entire host of allergies.

The atopic allergy usually begins at infancy. A rash on the face may be the first sign. The rash is accompanied by pronounced itching, and may ooze liquid.

A five-year-old youngster came into my office accompanied by both parents and two grandparents. The boy had gloves on his hands. Everybody talked at once. I got the picture without having to hear the words. These overly protective parents had gone through what their progeny was now suffering—atopic dermatitis, a frequently inherited tendency.

The parents had put gloves on the child to prevent him from scratching his chest. They also told how they had to literally overpower the child to keep him from scratching his body. They even had to tie him in his bed.

"Do something, Doctor," the grandparents pleaded.

The eczema was infected. It was oozing pus and had a bad odor. I prescribed cold baths of Aveeno, an oatmeal preparation that is very soothing. Kids love it. Aveeno baths should be taken two or three times a day, ten or fifteen minutes. The eczema begins to dry, and the edge is taken off the itching.

Tie children's hands and you infuriate them. It is an emotional disaster. The skin reacts unfavorably to emotional stress. It is far better to cut the child's fingernails, so there will be no possibility of infection from foreign matter under the nails.

After the child's skin began to dry, I prescribed an oral antihistamine and cortisone cream for his skin. I am not afraid of using cortisone injections for children, but I only use them for brief periods.

I remind parents of children with atopic eczema that these are extra-sensitive children, that they are usually much smarter than average, and highly motivated. Their eczema attacks occur at times of emotional stress, like examination time.

Emotions play an important part in atopic dermatitis. So we support these patients not only physically, but emotionally as well. Later, I will tell how biofeedback equipment can help atopic patients to relieve itching and control emotions.

Of course, atopic patients need to avoid common skin irritants, too. They may not be allergic to the wool in a wool sweater, but they react to the irritation of that rough material.

The quality of the fabric they wear should be smooth and non-irritating to their extra-sensitive skin.

Also, individuals prone to atopic disorders need to keep their distance from persons with herpes simplex. A cold sore can be "caught" through minimal contact, and the results can be very unfortunate. An atopic person with herpes simplex or herpes zoster can get the condition all over the body, and be very sick.

Youngsters with atopic dermatitis tendencies need to avoid physical and emotional stress. They can play at their usual games, but if they sweat, they will make their skin worse. They can play ball, swim, or do whatever they want to do. But they should pause to rest frequently. I don't ask my young patients to sit at home watching other kids play outside. They need to be active. But instead of riding a bike two hours, atopic children should cut the exercise to one hour—and cool off.

Youngsters with severe outbreaks of atopic dermatitis should be hospitalized. I feel that just getting these children away from an irritating environment helps in itself. Even getting them to go to live with a relative gets them away from the irritation or stress that they are having at home.

Breathing allergy, touching allergy, emotional allergy—all react favorably to a change in environment that separates the patient from the cause.

By the time youngsters reach adolescence, certainly by the time they reach adulthood, eczema is usually less of a problem.

I also see adults with eczema. If an adult has eczema, maybe it is just a small spot as on the hand. A history usually shows that although the atopic adult did not have eczema as a child, his or her parents did have it when they were young, and it is also probable that some of the patient's relatives have asthma, hayfever, migraine headaches, etc.—all atopic symptoms, albeit not on the skin.

One woman who had hand eczema had been to at least twelve doctors. She had tried everything, with no result. She was told that she was allergic to soap, so she was using soap substitutes. Her skin did not get better. When I diagnosed her condition as atopic dermatitis aggravated by emotional conditions, she readily admitted to an emotional crisis in her life. Tranquilizers and cortisone injections to make her more comfortable were the only treatments given. I told the women to be patient. Her skin improved immediately, and in several weeks the condition had cleared.

This chapter on allergies has been devoted largely to sleuthing techniques. I hope you never have to put on that detective badge.

Skin Mishaps from Sex, Insects, Poisons, or Injury

The skin you live in protects your vital organs and systems from the outside environment. This environment can be cold or hot, dry or wet, but the interior of your body remains at a fairly constant temperature and moistness.

There are many other goings on in the external environment that are inimical to our interior environment. These include encounters with other people, with animals, with plants, and with inanimate materials.

We can get bruises and black eyes from other people. Other people can also give us venereal disease. Our skin bears the brunt of encounters with biting animals such as spiders and insects. Many plants can poison our skin. The inanimate world threatens us with cuts, scrapes, burns, and bruises.

To keep our skin radiant, youthful, and vibrant, we need to minimize these harmful encounters with the outside environment, but when they do occur, we need to know how to handle such mishaps so as to minimize damage and permit the skin to rapidly restore itself to its high level of attractiveness.

Speaking of attractiveness, let's start with the sexual encounter.

Venereal Disease—Skin Touches Skin

The most common problem resulting from sexual encounters is herpes simplex. That's right—the common cold sore is a venereal disease. The word "venereal" comes from "Venus," the goddess of love.

Most venereal disease seems to have little to do with love relationships, more to do with passing sexual encounters.

The most prevalent venereal disease (second to herpes simplex), is gonorrhea; third is syphilis.

Herpes simplex is a virus. This virus can cause a skin problem. This skin problem can appear on both the regular skin and on mucous membrane skin, such as the lip of the mouth or the lip of the vagina. It can also be inside the mouth and inside the vagina.

Wherever the sore appears, herpes simplex is all produced by the same virus. But when the herpes virus is on the lip, it is called a cold sore. When the virus is on the penis or vagina, it is called venereal disease. One can become the other simply through oral sex.

Not so long ago, two types of herpes simplex were recognized. Type I always occurred above the waist. Type II always occurred below the waist. But now, with sexual activity apparently more permissive and diversified, the two types of herpes simplex virus have become interchangeable.

Today, if the virus is on the genitals we call it VD. "Well," you say, "my partner had a cold sore on the lip. Now I have one on the genitals. Does that mean I have VD but my sex partner doesn't?"

No, you both have venereal disease—more by "definition" than by lab tests. Because of the mix-up between Type I and Type II herpes simplex virus due to the mix-up in sexual techniques, the lab test is useless; and the above or below-the-belt definition gives way to whether or not the virus is sexually related. The spreading of the cold sore or herpes simplex by sexual contact—mouth to mouth or mouth to genitals—becomes the criterion for defining it as VD.

How is herpes simplex treated?

Herpes simplex is *not* treated with penicillin. Penicillin is anti-bacterial. It does not affect the virus.

Tetracycline and other antibiotics are also useless against the herpes simplex virus.

There are some vaccines in use in other countries that reduce the incidence of herpes simplex, both its frequency and severity. One vaccine was in use in the United States several years ago, but is not permitted now. This vaccine is still available in Germany and several other European countries.

Research is underway here that promises to produce some effective medication, but meanwhile. . . .

We treat herpes simplex venereal disease basically the same way that we treat herpes simplex cold sores, as described in the preceding chapter of this book. We use ice, cold packs, cortisone injections, liquid nitrogen, photo inactivation dyes, and chemicals to quiet down irritation.

To control the spread of herpes simplex venereal disease, it is advisable to get medical help for any cold sore-like lesion on the genitals, or any cold sore not on the genitals that might have been transmitted from the genitals.

Gonorrhea and Your Skin

Gonorrhea is defined as an infectious disease of the genitourinary tract, rectum, and cervix, caused by the *gonococcus* bacteria.

A man knows when he has contracted gonorrhea because he has a discharge from his penis—an urethral dripping—and he experiences burning and discomfort when urinating. Also, he finds it almost impossible to have sexual relations. Gonorrhea is almost always identified by the male patient.

However, the symptoms of gonorrhea are more subtle in the female, and usually go unnoticed. The female patient does not have the above symptoms.

One of the effects of gonorrhea in both sexes is sterility. The infected male can no longer impregnate, the infected female can no longer become pregnant.

The dermatologist has entered this picture more frequently in recent years, because the skin manifestations of gonorrhea seem to be increasing.

When gonorrhea is not treated, or when treatment by

penicillin or other antibacterial drugs is not effective, the bloodstream can be infected. This infection is usually transmitted to the skin, and red blisters or red sores form. Also, the infection can get into the joints and cause an arthritis.

Here there is no discrimination between the sexes as there is in the initial phase of gonorrhea. Both male and female can suffer the genital-blood-skin-joint cycle.

A woman, a divorcée in her thirties, came in with a skin problem. She showed me a mysterious red spot that had suddenly appeared on her arm. The spot was flat. I recognized it as a blood vessel that had become enlarged and then broken down—a possible sign of gonorrhea. I could find only a few such enlarged vessels. They would usually be more widespread, anywhere on the body. And the skin could blister.

The enlarged blood vessels could also be accompanied with fever, a sick feeling, pains, or arthritis.

This patient was getting off relatively easy, and prompt treatment helped. Prompt treatment also helped to prevent her recent sexual partners from spreading the disease, as they were told to contact their physicians if they had not already felt the discomfort, and done so.

Syphilis—Secret Sexual Scourge

The most prevalent venereal disease used to be syphilis. It is relatively uncommon now for a doctor to be asked to treat syphilis. Syphilis seems to be on the wane. But syphilis always has been an "undercover" agent.

The spirochete, the cause of syphilis, is a wiggly little organism that travels easily from skin to skin.

Once contracted, syphilis forms a painless sore on the skin. This sore heals in a few weeks. It is usually on the genitals, but it can be anywhere on the anatomy. The syphilitic sore feels hard and rubbery to the touch. The sore occurs when skin-to-skin contact is made. So it can be transmitted even without the sex act having been performed.

There is the case of a man who got syphilis on his toe. He was an avid bridge player, and had played "footsie" under the table with his partner, using his foot in intimate parts of her anatomy.

The usual place for the syphilis sore is on the penis. The sore favors places where there is a cut or scrape on the skin, but more typically it appears on mucous membranes, genitals, and lips. The sore can appear on the fingers, hands, nipples—anywhere that contact has occurred.

Because the sore, called a chancre, is not painful, and because it disappears in a couple of weeks, many cases of syphilis never get reported.

For the carrier of the secretive syphilis spirochete, the chancre is only the beginning. The little creature can be at the syphilitic's funeral; in fact, it could have caused the death. The spirochete eats away at vital organs, including heart and brain tissue.

Sometimes the patient is lucky—syphilis again surfaces on the skin a few weeks after the chancre disappears. Now it looks somewhat like a measles rash. It stays for a few weeks, and again goes away. The disappearance of this symptom again reassures most people, and they do nothing about it—until it is too late.

This rash is called "secondary" syphilis. The third phase can go in a number of directions—eye, heart, kidney, or brain. The rash has been the last observable symptom on the skin. From now on, the spirochete burrows internally, and may eventually cause insanity and death.

The treatment for syphilis is simple, fast and effective—penicillin.

Although there are strains of gonorrhea developing that require extra large doses of penicillin, or of some other stronger, more toxic antibiotic, no such developments have been noticed with the syphilis spirochete. Penicillin eradicates it.

So much for the skin-to-skin contact between people, and the not-so-lovable results of the so-called "loving relationship."

Bee Stings and Other Types of Insect Bites

In the animal world, the greatest problem comes from insect bites. Every one of us gets bitten many times during the year by one insect or another. Either we do not even know it, or at most, it causes us a few hours of itching, e.g., the mosquito bite.

However, thousands of people annually are stung by insects, and suffer severe—and sometimes fatal—reactions.

Why does one person forget a bee sting in a few hours, while another person suffers severe sickness? Until about forty years ago, this was believed to be due to the variations in bees. However, there has been a growing awareness of the role that allergic reactions play in people.

A study in 1958 showed that 94 percent of all the fatalities for the previous ten years due to the bites of venomous animals in the United States were from insects, snakes, and spiders, with bees and wasps accounting for about half of these.

Even fleas and mosquitoes can cause considerable local swelling in susceptible individuals. Allergic reactions have been reported from the bites of house flies, sand flies, and deerflies. And of course, chiggers and bedbugs make their presence known in no uncertain way.

There is a little known, easily obtainable product that provides practically immediate relief from bee and wasp stings: Adolph's Meat Tenderizer! (Thank you, Dr. Harry L. Arnold, Jr!) Meat tenderizer is a protein enzyme that helps the body protein to inactivate the toxin that gets into the skin. Mix a little Adolph's with some water to form a paste, and just place the paste on the bite. Keep the swollen area open and put ice on it, either indirectly or in a plastic bag. Take aspirin for the pain—aspirin is anti-inflammatory, so it cuts down on some the cause of that pain, too.

Do not probe the bite for the stinger. The skin rejects the stinger, and it comes out by itself.

A cold remedy like Contac can relieve discomfort, as it has an anti-histamine in it. Other products that offer similar relief, which you might have around the house, include Benadryl, Chlor-Trimeton, Pyribenzamine, and Periactin. These are antihistamines that can cut down on the itching and inflammation.

A cortisone product will relieve itching. You may have a recently obtained product around the house, which you used previously for an allergy.

Old-fashioned calamine lotion applied with a paint brush is also a reliever of insect-bite itching. Calamine is zinc oxide. It is pink and soothing. That indoor plant, aloe, is also soothing. Aloe helps burns, itching, and stings because of its anti-inflammatory effects, which are similar to the effects of cortisone.

Poison Ivy and Other Plant-Induced Rashes

Your druggist carries sprays that are helpful in relieving the discomfort of poison ivy and its urushiol cousins.

Calamine lotion or other topical preparations (externally applied) are also effective. Benzocaine, which provides a soothing effect, is the active ingredient in most of the spray preparations. Benzocaine has an anesthetic effect, but zirconium, a metal, may itself cause an irritation.

While Calamine is soothing, Caladryl, in my opinion, should not be used. Caladryl is a combination of Calamine and Benadryl. The latter is an antihistamine. Antihistamines are fine when taken internally, but when placed on the skin, they can themselves cause a contact dermatitis.

The safest and cheapest treatment for rashes is water. Cold compresses applied to the inflamed area are soothing.

This does not mean soaking the affected skin in water, like putting your foot or hand in a bucket or sink. This works against the skin's own healing process. Wet a towel, handkerchief, or bandage. The colder the water, the better. Ice water is fine. Wet the compress frequently. Keep it on for a few minutes to an hour for good results.

Milk can also be used for your compress. The protein in milk has a soothing effect. Use half milk, half water.

Poison ivy goes away. It is hard to realize that while you have it. So you listen to neighbors, Grandma and Cousin Joe. One might say, "use vaseline," another, "butter," or a third, "salt." Rather than play favorites, you put on all three. Result: complications.

The less you do for plant-induced rashes, the better.

If you have an aloe plant, you have a homegrown source of skin relief. Break off a tip of one of the leaves. Squeeze the oily substance directly onto the poison ivy or other contact dermatitis. Aloe has an excellent soothing effect, without any risk of irritation. Don't try other plants.

THE UBIQUITOUS URUSHIOLS	
Common Names	*Scientific Names*
Mango "King of the fruits" "Apple of the tropics"	*Mangifera indica*
Poison Ivy Common poison ivy, poison creeper, markweed	*Rhus radicans*
Oakleaf Poision Ivy Eastern oakleaf Poison Ivy	*Rhus diversilobum*
Poison Sumac Swamp sumac, poison elder, poison dogwood	*Rhus vernix*
Poison Oak Western poison oak, yeara	*Rhus toxicodendron*
Lacquer Tree Japanese lacquer tree	*Rhus vernicifera*
Cashew Nut Shell Oil Cashew oil	*Anacardium occidentale*
Indian Marking Nut Dhobie (washerman) itch	*Bella gutti*
Rengas Tree Black varnish tree	*Anacardium melanorrhoe*
Ginkgo Tree Maidenhair tree	*Ginkgo biloba*

Distribution	*Modes of Contact*
Hawaii, California Florida, India, Central America, Mediterranean	Direct—plant or fruit to skin. or Indirect—animal fur, door handles, clothing, particles in air, tools, mosquitoes, golf clubs, fishing tackle, etc.
USA (but not Southwest) Canada, Mexico, Taiwan, Western China	
Southeastern USA	
Southeastern USA	
Pacific Coast USA	
Japan, China, India	Voodoo dolls, swizzle sticks, resins, mucilages, wood boxes, bracelets, bar rails.
India, Africa, Central America, East Indies	Printer's ink, electrical insulation.
India, Malaya	Laundry marking ink
Malaya	Furniture, wood, carvings
Southeastern USA, China Japan, Europe	Soaps, cosmetics, Oriental lacquerware, stepping on seeds.

Itching, the plague of contact dermatitis, can be relieved by taking aspirin by mouth.

Cold water and aspirin. This is not very satisfying professional advice to patients who visit a dermatologist.

"I did not come here, Doc, just to get cold water."

What do you do for the patient who insists on instant relief by some magical means? Aveeno is my answer. I have them buy Aveeno at the pharmacy. Aveeno is an oatmeal preparation. For large areas, you can throw a handful of it into the bath water and sit in the Aveeno bath for awhile. For smaller areas, follow the instructions on the package. Aveeno forms a soothing film on the surface of the skin, and helps to heal it faster.

But to you I say, cold water.

In the previous chapter, we talked about the "ubiquitous urushiols." On pages 118-119 is a chart showing the many common locations and modes of contact of the ubiquitous urushiols. Below, are drawings of poison ivy, oak, sumac, and their poisonous cousins.

The ubiquitous urushiols.

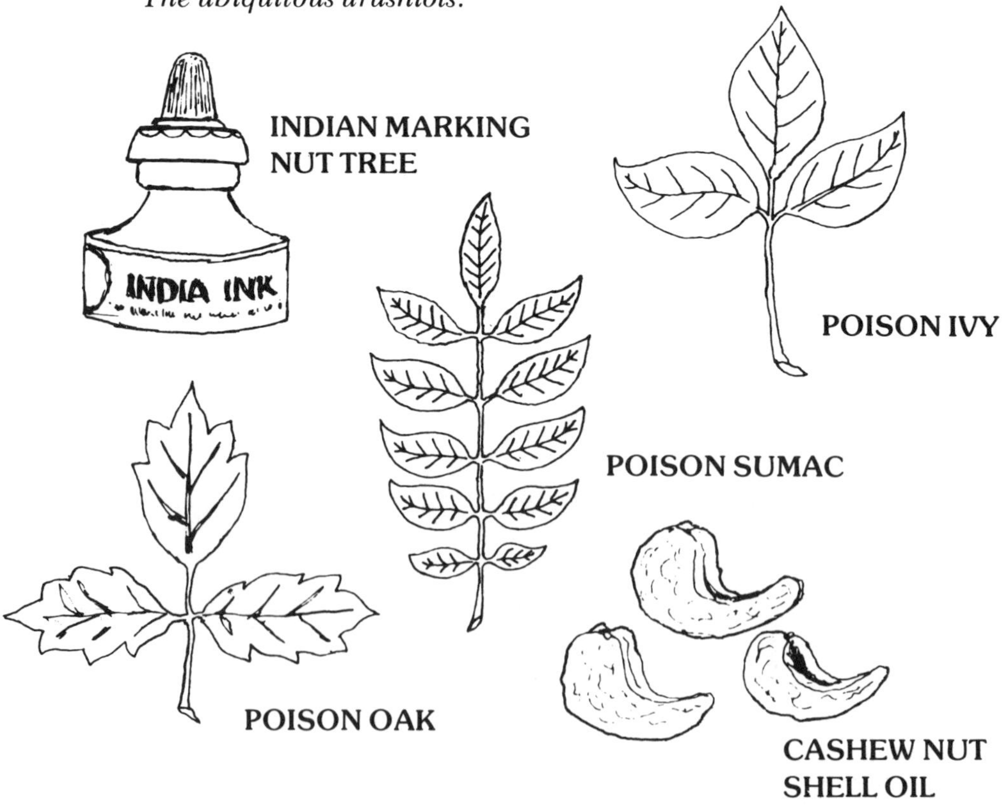

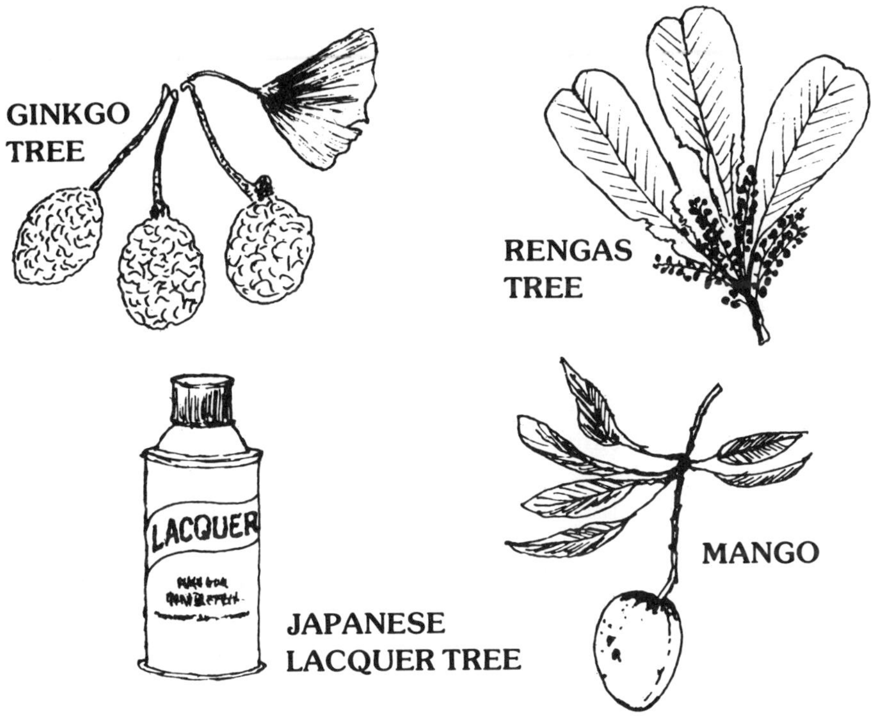

Burns—How to Play Them Cool

Burns are by far the most frequent means by which the inanimate world causes injury to skin. We have already covered the way the sun can burn us, and how to treat such burns. Now what do we do when we are scalded in the kitchen, or burned by a flame or by a chemical?

Skin enzymes break down when skin is burned. The enzyme breakdown produces a fluid. This fluid forms blisters.

Many people are frightened by this fluid. It is just ordinary fluid. It is not contagious. It does not spread from here to there.

Most small burns (such as on the back of the hands) are not serious enough to warrant a visit to your doctor. Just do not tamper with the blister. Do not pop the blister; play it cool. Just let the burn alone. The blister will heal.

Problems that arise from small burns are usually due to putting something on to hasten the healing. I repeat—play it cool. If you must put something on the burn, use a cold water compress.

A cold water compress has a soothing effect on a burn and it cannot harm the skin. This does not mean soaking the hand in water, as I mentioned in connection with insect bites. Soaking the burn causes the skin to become super saturated—mushy and soggy—and healing bogs down. Use a washcloth or handkerchief dropped in ice-cold water. This permits the water to evaporate, cooling the burn as it does.

How about coconut oil, butter, or other lubricants? They will do no good at all. Lubricants do not reduce the enzymatic breakdown. They do not reduce the blisters. Lubricants serve no purpose at all. In fact, in my opinion, any oil makes burns worse.

A woman came to my office with a burned foot. A housewife, she had knocked against the handle of a pot sticking over the edge of the range, and had spilled boiling soup on her foot.

Had she "cooled it," and done nothing but put cold compresses on the burned foot, that would have been the end of the story. But the woman put Caladryl and butter on her burns. The Caladryl caused contact dermatitis, and the sticky, oily butter complicated the situation.

Fluid seeps more readily into the lower part of the body, due to gravity. The woman had a great deal of oozing from her burned foot, and itching from the contact dermatitis. Three days later, when she came in, she had an infection. The infection was pussy and foul smelling. The patient also had red streaks leading up her leg from the infected area, indicating that she had what is commonly known as blood poisoning. The infection was going into the rest of her body. She had a fever.

We treated the woman with antibiotics, got her off her feet, and prescribed nothing else except cold compresses. Whenever you have an infection in the lower extremities, elevate them. Sleep with your pillow under your feet, instead of under your head. Sit with your feet up. This reduces swelling by simple fluid dynamics. Within a few days, the woman's foot healed, leaving a small scar to remind her—next time, cool it.

Most dermatologists will agree that the less you put on acute dermatitis burns, the better.

Some people prefer the feel of warm water to the feel of cold water. When they ask me whether they could use a hot compress instead of a cold compress, I say go ahead. But when you take off the hot compress, put on a cold compress. The cold compress stops the sweat formation, and slows up the fluid accumulation after the burn.

Avoid sun exposure after a burn. The sun can cause the burn to become darker or lighter than the surrounding skin. If the burn is over a sizeable area, and is oozing or dripping, keep it covered. A small finger burn should be kept uncovered.

If a blister gets very large, you can release the fluid by heating a pin in a flame to partially sterilize it, and then gently pricking the blister with the sterilized pin. After you "pop" the blister, do not remove it. The roof of a blister is the best possible "bandage" you can have. It flattens on to the burn, forms a dressing, then peels off by itself when its job is done.

If you peel the roof of the blister off, or pick at it, you run the risk of infection—a high risk.

If the blister does become infected, an externally applied antibiotic is usually an effective treatment. An antibiotic in a cream form is better than an antibiotic ointment.

The difference between a cream and an ointment is often important to know. Both creams and ointments are salves. Salve is a general term. An ointment is greasy, like Vaseline. A cream is oil-water suspension; cold cream is an example. The big difference is the oily or greasy base of the ointment. Where you do not wish to put oil on the skin, as in the case of burns, you use a cream. Your antibiotic now is an antibiotic cream.

Peroxide is a good home treatment for a skin infection. Peroxide does not burn or stick, and it is easy to apply. Peroxide adds oxygen to the affected area, and thus accelerates healing.

Iodine is effective, but it burns. Even decolorized and weakened iodine is quite irritating.

PHisoHex is excellent for infected burns. It used to be sold over the counter, but now it is sold by prescription only. PHisoHex is safe to use. It is an antibiotic soap. For generations PHisoHex was used with no problems, but then there were instances of it being used on babies with toxic effects. This had occurred because too much PHisoHex had been used and not washed off, so it was absorbed by the babies' skin. PHisoHex can be toxic if left on the skin. If your doctor prescribes PHisoHex, use it: it is perfectly safe used according to his directions. PHisoHex kills bacteria.

Zephiran is another antibacterial cleansing product. It comes in solution form, and is sold over the counter.

Is Your Burn First, Second, or Third-Degree?

The severity of burns is measured by two factors. The first is area. It is believed that burns over 75 percent of the body's surface are almost always fatal. Medical people have a quick way of measuring this, giving each part of the body a fraction like one-ninth for an arm, etc. When 50 percent of the body's surface is affected by the burn, it is touch and go.

The second factor by which the severity of a burn is measured has to do with the intensity of the burn. This in turn is a measure of the temperatures involved, and the contact of the skin with that temperature.

Because the damage to the skin resulting from a burn falls into three general categories, those categories have been given numbers to identify the degree of the burn—first, second or third-degree burns.

A first-degree burn is a superficial burn. It is basically a redness of the skin with some swelling and pain.

A second-degree burn is when the skin is blistered and red.

A third-degree burn is when the damage is deeper. The burn goes below the epidermis, or outer skin, and affects the dermis, or middle layers of skin, and even the subcutaneous tissue, the deepest layer of skin.

Cuts or burns that go below the outer layer of skin can cause bleeding and scarring if they reach the blood system. Fat globules come through when you cut or burn the deepest layers of skin. You can see these as yellow droplets.

A third-degree burn is a candidate for immediate medical attention, even if it is just on a finger.

First and second-degree burns on a small area can be handled at home as described above, but over a large area they, too, should get professional care. How large is large? If a significant portion of an arm is burned, by all means see your doctor.

The body can lose a significant amount of serous fluid through a burned area. This loss of serous fluid, as well as infection, can be the danger factor. One of the first treatments supplied in serious burn cases is the restoration of body fluid intravenously.

In the case of serious burns demanding immediate medical attention, wrap the affected area with a wet handkerchief or pillowcase, as a cold compress. A dry compress can damage the tissue when removed. The application of peroxide to a temporary dressing also facilitates the removal of the bandage.

Easing the Discomfort of Prickly Heat

Sometimes the inanimate environment provides a combination of characteristics that affects the skin. The temperature does not have to be extreme, but when warmth is combined with humidity, some skin may react with what has become known as prickly heat.

Prickly heat is a common problem, not just limited to children, but causing discomfort to adults also. Prickly heat comes from sweat retention. If the skin becomes soggy and moist, the sweat does not emerge from the skin but gets trapped, forming tiny sweat blisters.

Sweat blisters may be filled with clear fluid, or the blisters may be red, due to the tiny blood vessels enlarging in this area. A mixture of blood and perspiration will also produce red blisters.

Common locations for sweat blisters are under the breasts, armpits, and groin. These are places where skin rubbing up against skin makes for moisture.

Can you guess what your skin would like to have you do for prickly heat? Right—apply cold water. Cold water quiets down the sweating. Wearing less clothing or more aerated types of clothing helps cut down sweating, too. A man should wear loose boxer-type shorts instead of the closer fitting jockey-type shorts.

Cool air is soothing to prickly heat. In your home, hook up an electric fan, and let the cool air soothe the irritated areas, spreading your legs or elevating your arms to expose the affected skin.

Infants get prickly heat mostly because of diapers, and what goes on inside diapers.

A mother brought in her six-month-old infant dressed in a suit that covered the wrists and ankles. The only part of the infant that showed was the head, covered by a tight-fitting woolen hat.

Besides having diaper rash, the child had prickly heat all over, and was running a fever. Merely by taking the clothing off to examine the child, I had already begun the treatment.

I told the mother that the excessive clothing was causing the condition. It is practically impossible to talk mothers out of using rubber pants over the baby's diapers—Pampers would be better—so I usually suggest changing the diaper more frequently.

Cooling the child off, including the use of a cool bath, would end the condition. Aveeno—that oatmeal preparation we already mentioned—in the bath makes it soothing.

Some people say that cornstarch is good for prickly heat. I do not like to use cornstarch, because it is a nutrient for yeast and can cause a fungus problem.

Even talcum powder can be an irritation to the skin. Recent microscopic examinations of talc have revealed that this substance has sharp edges. Skin rubbed with most talcum powders has actually been irritated—as if the skin had been rubbed with sandpaper. Only a very fine talcum powder—such as Johnson's Baby Powder—can be soothing instead of irritating. Zeasorb is a natural product made from corncobs or husks. Zeasorb does not have sharp edges. So Zeasorb is an over-the-counter powder that you can use safely and soothingly for prickly heat.

Cuts that Bleed Profusely

Inanimate environment sometimes takes the form of paring knives, scissors, and lawn mowers. These servants of man can suddenly become his tormentors. Result: deep cuts of the skin we live in. Blood, gore, and maybe even an amputated finger tip.

This is going to be a short discourse, because you are probably well practiced in handling superficial cuts, especially if you are a man who shaves.

On the other hand, the more serious cuts that bleed profusely you are not going to "handle" at all, except perhaps for some first aid—our present subject.

The best thing you can do to help yourself in case of a deep cut that bleeds profusely is to apply pressure. Take a piece of cotton and press the cotton on the wound. Bleeding will stop with pressure.

If the wound is so large that you cannot put pressure on the entire area, and if it is on an arm or a leg, you might have to use a tourniquet. Tourniquet-making is taught in first aid classes, remember? You tie a handkerchief loosely above the wound; then place a stick in the loop, and tighten the tourniquet by twisting. This cuts off the blood supply to the entire limb, so the tourniquet must be loosened frequently, or there is a risk of gangrene—with subsequent loss of limb.

If you cut off a piece of a finger, the tip of a nose, or any part of your body, don't throw the lost part away. Wrap it in a moist handkerchief and bring it to the treatment area with you. Plastic surgeons are skilled at sewing lost parts of the body back on.

A twenty-six-year-old man in California recently had his scalp complete ripped off when his long hair got caught in a spinning drive shaft of his truck, after he crawled under the truck to make an adjustment. Six surgeons worked in teams to reconnect every small blood vessel; the task required tedious surgery with the aid of a microscope. This man became the first person in the country to have his scalp sewn back on.

Black-and-Blue Marks

It might be argued that more bruises occur as a result of human contact than as a result of contact with inanimate objects, but I place that black eye in this section out of deference to the person who claims, "I bumped into a door."

Bruises and black-and-blue marks are traumatizations of the skin, with probable subsurface bleeding.

The greatest risk comes from you—from your putting something on the abrasion to cause a contact dermatitis. Yes, most common house cures for these simple cuts and bruises are "worse than the disease."

Use cold water on the bruise.

Take Vitamin C.

You already know about the soothing, healing benefits of cold water, but let me say a word about why I recommend Vitamin C.

Vitamin C taken orally heals connective tissues. These connective tissues are what are damaged in bruises. Vitamin C accelerates the healing. Vitamin C does nothing applied to the skin. It must be swallowed.

We get some bruises to treat in the office, but by and large those visits are unnecessary. People panic. They fear the worst. This does not help the body in its natural healing responses.

Fear, tension, and anxiety are the doctor's opponents, no matter what needs to be cured.

One woman came into my office hysterical. She would tell the nurse nothing. She had to see me. She caused such a disturbance in the waiting room, that they ushered her right into a treatment room. She was moaning and sobbing when I saw her, barely able to tell me the problem; she was caring for a burned person in her family, and had accidentally touched the oozing part! She showed me her hands. There was nothing there. I did notice that the nails were bitten. She was the nervous type.

Nothing I said about the burned person's fluid being harmless seemed to get through to her. Her agitation only seemed to get worse. Finally, I gave her a mild antihistamine injection, purely for its sedative effect. The injection calmed her down a bit. I asked her to call me that night to tell me how she felt. That night she reported that the injection was marvelous. "The infection is all gone, Doctor!"

P.S.: This woman returned many times in the future with other crises—all imagined, like delusions of parasites. The samples of "parasites" she brought in included lint, belly button fuzz, and dust particles. Once, she brought in samples of "bugs" that she had pulled off her skin, all captured neatly and lined up on scotch tape. Under examination, the "bugs" proved to be blackheads, hair, and lint. I see many hypochondriac patients like this. Even if you let them look through the microscope, they refuse to accept the truth. These people have emotional, not skin, problems. But I always treat them—mostly with placebos, concern, and "TLC" (tender, loving care).

One nineteen-year-old secretary whom I first treated for a herpes simplex on her lip came back in a week or so with a mild yeast infection on the corners of her mouth. Two weeks later, she came back with a very mild infection on her finger. She had one problem after another.

At first, I thought this patient had an immunological problem, or was rundown, or maybe diabetic. So we checked with blood tests. Everything was O.K. This young secretary's problem turned out to be loneliness! Her body was actually "creating" these problems, so she could see me. This is great for a doctor's ego, but who needs such "headaches?" I referred her back to her family doctor.

The Most Intelligent Organ in Your Body

The brain is the seat of intelligence. But intelligence manifests itself through every cell, every organ, every system.

I vote for the skin as the most intelligent part of the body. The heart is fantastic: it pumps away in just the right manner. But the skin is even more fantastic.

The skin gets thicker if it has to get thicker, as on the bottom of the foot.

If the skin has to be thinner for sensation, it is thin, as on the genitals.

The skin develops hair for protection against the elements, including sun damage. The skin creates more pigmentation to protect itself from the sun's rays.

The skin activates its sweat glands to lower the body temperature when necessary.

The skin blushes with anger to make your opponent afraid of your redness.

The skin bristles its hair to make the hair stand on end—another attempt to scare the opponent.

Doctor and patient probably do too much for the skin. The skin probably knows better than either doctor or patient what to do for itself most of the time. We overtreat the skin while nature is already doing what needs to be done—forming callouses around irritations, cooling them with fluid, ejecting foreign matter from the body.

Your skin is naturally healthy. I admire skin that has color to it; that has just the right moisture; that has other radiant signs of a high level of good heatlh.

This is skin that is being permitted to do its "own thing"—be healthy—free of our interference through unhealthy food, attitudes, or living habits.

The external environment creates wear and tear on the skin. The environment is a factor in aging. But as we examine aging in the next chapter, we need to include the internal environment—mental and physical—in our examination as well.

How You Can Change Aging to Youthful Skin

Periodically, mankind seems to launch a search for the fountain of youth. We appear to be on such a safari right now, as scientists journey into the depths of the molecule to study its genetic secrets in the hope of controlling the aging process.

In dermatology, we are directing our explorations against aging to ways of restoring youthful skin. You might say that this is a superficial approach—limited only to the skin we live in. But beauty's domain is the skin; and beauty, though it be only skin deep, goes quite deeply indeed into the entire motivation for the search for youth.

This chapter is about recapturing a youthful appearance. It is directed to both men and women. However, there are two reasons why more women will find it useful to them than will men. One, masculine attractiveness depends less on "baby" skin than feminine attractiveness. Two, the process of shaving encourages new skin to replace old skin at a faster rate.

This replacement of old skin with new is going on all the time. However, the process slows up. Skin begins to show more old cells.

To change this older look—the wrinkles, the brown spots, the crowsfeet and seams—to a fresh new face takes "processing."

This processing can be accomplished by your dermatologist with your help; or it can be done by specialists using particular processes—such as plastic surgery, or cosmetic clinics and spas. We will discuss these latter special approaches later in this chapter, but first let us examine how you and your dermatologist can take ten or twenty years off your appearance.

Rehabilitating Skin "Worn" by Life

Life makes its mark on us. Life "gets" to us, inside and out. But it is on the outside, or the skin, that we see the "scars" of life's trials and tribulations visibly. We call these scars aging.

You can improve your good looks by removing these signs of aging, especially from your face. It is quite easy to make noticeable improvements. These improvements do not cost much. You may already have in your home the necessary materials to make them. Nor does skin care take much time, or necessarily require a visit to your dermatologist's office.

When you improve your skin, you improve your physical appearance. When you improve your physical appearance, you improve your psyche. So improve the outer you, and you improve the inner you.

Mrs. Mary L. from the Deep South, seventy-two years old, looked every one of those years when she came to see me. Her son-in-law, a physician, had recommended the visit, not because there was anything wrong with Mary's skin, but because Mary was feeling depressed about her years.

She had multiple blackheads, dark spots, and white bumps on her skin. It was old, dry skin. It gave her an aged look. Also, she had excess hair on her face.

I suggested a program of treatment to Mary that included the following:

An abrasive soap

A blackhead remover

Moisturizing preparations

Electrolysis

By using the abrasive soap, Mary gave herself a mini- dermabrasion. She rubbed off the top layers of skin. Lava soap is cheap and effective, but there are more elegant soaps that have a fragrance, and are not expensive. These soaps include Komex, Pernox, Brasivol, and an abrasive pad that has come out recently called Buf Puf. Buf Puf is an abrasive sponge.

Mary used one of the fragrant abrasive soaps several times a day; she purposely irritated her skin slightly, causing the top layer to shed off like a sunburn. Healthier skin grew in from underneath.

Mary obtained a LaCross blackhead remover, which was described earlier in the treatment for acne. Every day, Mary spent a few minutes removing blackheads.

After that, she began to use the moisturizing preparations on her face. These were not greasy or sticky. These preparations hydrated the skin without adding oil. These moisturizing treatments were to smooth out the wrinkles that Mary had. These wrinkles were due to irregular folds in the skin caused by cumulative sun damage to the connective tissue over the years. Fibers in the skin were lost, costing the skin some of its elasticity. More about these preparations in our next chapter.

Then Mary went to an electrologist, a technician who removes hair with an electric needle. She had this hair on her upper lip, due to the increase of male hormones that comes with aging.

Electrolysis was probably the most expensive part of her treatment. Three or four visits cost her about seventy-five dollars. But what a difference! The facial hair was gone. She looked so much more feminine from this alone. There are devices sold over the counter to remove hair, but I do not recommend them.

Once Mary had reduced the number of cysts and blackheads on her face, induced new skin, moisturized her face, and removed facial hair, she went to a beauty parlor and had her hair done in a more youthful style.

When Mary returned to my office for her next visit, she looked easily twenty years younger. She bubbled with energy and enthusiasm. I could feel that her psyche was just released from the prison we call old age. "Norman," she said with a broad smile and an even broader southern accent, "Ah love you."

How to Erase Years from Your Face

A word first to remind you that we are not turning back the years. You cannot fool Mother Nature. She knows your age. You can only fool those who look at you. You can do this by altering the skin "language." Your skin "telegraphs" your age. Its message does not always correspond to your chronological age.

A thirty-five-year-old woman can look fifty because of what her skin has been through. What we are doing is working with this skin language, so that the telegraphed message comes across instead as a fifty-year-old looking thirty-five.

Wrinkles are the most common "words" in this skin language. Get rid of lines, folds, crows feet, and seams, and the answer to "how old?" comes through loud and clear as "young!"

We can remove surface wrinkles in several ways. One way of removing surface wrinkles is by chemically peeling them off. The chemical usually used is phenol. We can also use acids. We can also scrape wrinkles off with dermabrasion,.or freeze them off with cryosurgery. Let's examine these alternatives from the point of view of:

Minimum of discomfort involved

Minimum of time involved

Maximum effectiveness

Let's start with methods that you can use yourself at home, without necessarily seeing a doctor.

There is a process known as epibrasion. It is done by you with a Buf Puf. The Buf Puf is gentle and mild, yet effective. It is just an abrasive sponge. You rub your face with a Buf Puf two or three times a day for a few days, and you can begin to see the results. Discomfort is minimal, time is minimal, but effectiveness is quite a bit more than minimal, depending on the original condition and your conscientiousness in use of the Buf Puf.

Abrasive soaps are also useful in removing old skin, wrinkles, and acne scars. One abrasive soap is Brasivol. Brasivol is available in fine, medium, and rough textures. You begin with the fine soap, removing the most superficial of age signs. Then you switch to medium, going deeper, and finally, you attack wrinkles with rough Brasivol. These soaps are available without prescription.

There are prescription preparations that both lighten the skin and peel the skin. One of these is not yet available for this purpose at this writing, but should be shortly. It is a Vitamin A acid, similar to a prescription preparation currently available for treating acne. This substance also contains a depigmenting solution, hydroquinone, and a low dose of cortisone. Off come senile spots and keratoses, while at the same time the skin is made a bit smoother. Watch for this product.

Lubricating the skin is another approach to rejuvenating the skin. However, there are right ways and wrong ways to lubricate. Unfortunately, most people use the wrong ways.

Greasing the skin does not get rid of wrinkles. Wrinkles are folds in the surface of the skin due to changes in the collagen or connective tissue below the surface of the skin. Nothing you put on the skin affects the connective tissue where wrinkles start.

There are wrinkle-removing creams, which when applied after the face is washed with cold water, will serve to "seal" in this water, causing the skin to retain water—the real moisturizer—rather than oil. Skin so moisturized shows the wrinkles less.

One of these over-the-counter anti-wrinkle preparations is Formula 405. Do not confuse this with Formula 409, an entirely different product for a different purpose (a househould cleanser), and manufactured by a different company. Formula 405 is an anti-wrinkle lubricant.

Other easily available anti-wrinkle creams are Carmol, Aquacare HP and Lacticare. These, and other related products, contain urea. Urea is not related to uric acid or urine. Urea helps retain fluid in the skin. So urea both moisturizes and lubricates, diminishing the visibility of wrinkles.

When you stop using any of these preparations, their effects are no longer apparent because the wrinkles are still basically there, and have been right along. Once you stop the treatments, you revert in appearance to your original wrinkled look.

Most people use these anti-wrinkle products twice a day. They are just as effective on the hands, chest, and other parts of the body where you wish wrinkles to be less in evidence. No discomfort, a little time, and some minor effectiveness.

If you still have wrinkles and other signs of old age that you want to reduce, better phone your dermatologist for a consultation appointment.

Professional Techniques to Restore the Youthful Look

Cryosurgery—the freezing process we discussed for acne and other skin problems—can be used to peel off the top layers of the skin. With these top layers of the skin go many of the signs of aging. When new skins grows back, it is young skin that "telegraphs" a younger look.

For white skin or light skin, cryosurgery is quite effective. However, for dark skin such as Negro skin or Oriental skin, there is a chance of hyperpigmentation. The skin can become darker.

This is the procedure for cryosurgery.

First, the face skin is frozen lightly, and there is fine peeling of the skin. This is repeated several times, varying from a total of three to six treatments, one layer of the facial skin at a time, until the whole face, forehead, and perhaps part of the neck has been given several such fine peelings.

If the patient is not thoroughly satisfied after a few treatments, I discontinue the cryosurgery. I always tell my patients not to expect cryosurgery to make the face "baby bottom" smooth. However, they should expect an improvement, perhaps 50 to 60 percent.

Those who are satisfied with this amount of improvement find that cryosurgery is relatively free of discomfort, that it is not incapacitating in any way, except that the face is not "presentable" to the public for a few days after each treatment.

If the change is not dramatic enough, and if the cryosurgery is ended, the patient can still choose to go into a more intensive treatment—dermabrasion.

Dermabrasion is done in the doctor's office. It can be by a plastic surgeon or by a dermatologist.

First, the patient is given a pre-operation pill, to cut down on the pain and on stress. Prior to coming in the patient has shampooed his hair and washed his face, and is told to be prepared for several hours in the doctor's office.

The patient lies down on a treatment table. His face is sprayed with ethyl chloride, a refrigerant. Ethyl chloride freezes the skin, making it hard. An inch at a time, the skin is literally scraped off. Dermabrasion is a bloody, messy procedure. There is less pain that you might think, but dermabrasion is still an uncomfortable, lengthy procedure, lasting two hours. Even the walls and ceiling of the doctor's office can get splattered with blood and skin.

After dermabrasion, the patient is incapacitated for about ten days. Dermabrasion patients have crusts and scabs on the skin for at least five days—and oozing of fluid. Bandages are applied to the skin. The face is actually "mummified" with dressings. Some patients are not able to return to school or occupation for two or three weeks following the operation, and even then are still not completely "healed." Usually, the patients come in with somebody to drive them home, as they will be drowsy after the operation. They return once or twice on the following days to have the dressing changed.

Of course, you can make dermabrasion a localized procedure. The more local, the less messy. Acne scarring and wrinkles can be targeted. The most common problem area for older women is around the mouth, where wrinkling is prevalent due largely to hormone changes, and there is a great deal of both dermabrasion and cryosurgery being performed now just for that localized aging problem.

Dermabrasion is sometimes called "the sandpaper operation." Indeed, a type of sterile sandpaper was originally used for this operation. Today, diamond fraises or abrasive wheels are used.

Medical plans usually consider dermabrasion as a strictly cosmetic procedure, so it is not covered by medical insurance. But you can deduct dermabrasion from your tax computations as a medical expense. I personally prefer cryosurgery to dermabrasion, not only because it is cleaner, faster, and easier on both doctor and patient, but also because I can control pigmentation better with liquid nitrogen. Abrasion irritates the pigmentation-producing cells called melanocytes, sometimes causing the skin to become darker in spots.

Both systems—cryosurgery and dermabrasion—are only as

good as your follow-up care. This boils down to simply staying out of the sun.

The sun causes wrinkles, and all the sandpapering and freezing will be for naught if you do not protect your new skin from this aging agent.

If you are subject to sun damage, you should know about another way of treating wrinkled skin—with 5-FU (five fluorouracil). This is a prescription cream used to get rid of cancer and pre-cancer on the skin. 5-FU is easy to use. The patient applies it at home, twice a day for three weeks.

I consider 5-FU a very effective preparation for the wrinkles that accompany aging. Be forewarned though, you will be unsightly for four to six weeks. Usually, you treat a small portion of the skin first, like a portion of the face or a small patch on the forehead. Then you see how you respond, and can decide to treat larger areas.

Or, you can throw in the sponge and decide to go in for plastic surgery. If you do, make up your mind that even in this "ultimate" procedure, you are seeking not a *young* face but a *younger* face. Plastic surgery is performed by a surgeon—usually in a hospital, where the stay can be one to three weeks, depending on the size of the operation, medical complications, and healing capacity of the patient.

Preventive Home Exercises to Slow Skin Aging

As I said before, working from the outside in does not get at the cause of wrinkling. Connective tissue below the epidermis is where the problem resides. Muscles become loose. You tighten them by special facial exercises.

For instance, wrinkles under the chin and at the lower jowl area can be helped by sticking your bottom lip out and holding it in that position for ten seconds, and also by lying in bed on your back, with your head hanging over the edge, and then opening and closing your mouth slowly for a few minutes.

To tighten horizontal lines under your chin at the top of your neck, stick out your tongue as far as it can go and curl it up. Hold it there for a few seconds, and then repeat a few times.

Similar exercises were put in book form* by their Hollywood originator, Mrs. Senta Maria Runge, in 1961, and are still widely practiced.

These exercises are good preventive "medicine." They are good wrinkle removal and lessening procedures. And they are good rehabilitation procedures after plastic surgery, to prolong the absence of wrinkles and folds.

There are many skin-rejuvenating processes that are making a name for themselves. Most of them are types of chemical peeling. Doctor Ronald Bennett, founder of the World Health Center in Los Angeles, uses a system he calls "exodermy." Other doctors with systems based on the same principle are conducting clinics in Mexico, Bermuda, and several European countries. Costs can run from one to several thousand dollars—many times the cost of cryosurgery. Skin rejuvenating treatments often include exercises, special foods, and relaxation therapy.

Hormones And Estrogen Creams As Rejuvenators

There are now a number of creams on the market that can be applied to the face and neck and promise a new youthful exuberance and elasticity to the skin. These are the hormone and estrogen creams.

An ounce bottle of this cream can cost about thirty dollars. The reason for this expensive price is that hormones are not easily produced in quantity for laboratory use.

Personally, I do not see these creams as doing any better at improving skin appearance than the cheaper urea products I mentioned before.

Hormone creams work better in vaginal areas. Older women get so-called atrophy of the vagina—dryness and cracking. This condition responds quite well to applications of hormone creams.

Royal jelly, queen bee jelly, and other "natural" jellies, together with pH creams, do not really do too much. For instance, the pH factor of the skin is self-correcting, unless you

---

**Face Lifting by Exercise*, Allegro Publishing Co., Los Angeles, California.

have some major metabolic disease such as uremia or diabetes or severe thyroid disease. Healthy people do not need to supply these substances to their skin.

There is nothing harmful about using "organic" creams. If it makes you feel good to put peach or cucumber creams on your face, then it is good for you to do it. If you like the way a "natural" product smells, tastes, or feels, use it.

A Fibrin Treatment for the Scars of Time

About twenty years ago a Boston doctor, A. S. Spangler (now deceased), devised a system of smoothing over wrinkles and scarred areas of skin by using a fibrin foam-injection method.

Fibrin is a blood constitutent. It is used in the procedure by making a small cut near a scar or certain type of wrinkle and injecting the fibrin under the skin. Thus implanted, the fibrin fills out the scar and makes it more flush with the skin surface. Fibrin does the same with a certain type of deep line or wrinkle.

This procedure is not yet approved by the Federal Drug Administration. It is perfectly safe, as fibrin is a natural constituent of blood. So the procedure is little more than a blood transfusion. But fibrin implantation does not produce the reaction sometimes produced in blood transfusions due to type of blood. Fibrin is not typed. It is common to all blood types. FDA approval may be already granted by the time you read this.

Both plastic surgeons and dermatologists will be eligible to do fibrin treatments, once approved.

Due to its limited application, fibrin implantation will probably never become as widely used as face lifting or other rejuvenating procedures. However, fibrin implantation is so simple and effective, that it will be a standard method one day in the near future for treating larger, crater-like scars from acne or chickenpox. These scars can be made inconspicuous by fibrin treatment to the point where any remaining blemish can be covered with cosmetics.

Also quite successfully treated with fibrin are the so-called "undulating scars," where there are no sharply defined borders and an irregular floor depth. Undulating scars are brought level with the surrounding skin with fibrin, and practically disappear. The same is true of "icepick" scars.

Novocaine is usually provided as a local anesthesia in fibrin treatments. The procedure is done gradually with a number of short treatments over a period of a few weeks. Unsightliness is at a minimum. At a minimum, too, are discomfort and periods of disability.

The fibrin treatment is reminiscent of silicone injections. Silicone injections began in Japan and Europe as liquid injections. There were some bad aftereffects. The liquid caused irritation. Sometimes it traveled from where it was injected—as for breast enlargement—to other parts of the body less able to tolerate it. Even in the breast, the silicone settled to the dependent part of the breast, where it frequently caused infection because of impurities.

If the woman had breast nodules, silicone increased the chances of developing breast cancer, because you could not feel through palpation with the fingers whether these were silicone or cancer nodules. Later, this liquid method was improved by using hard, rubber-like balls of silicone, but the balls proved quite unnatural to the look and touch.

Today, silicone is used more safely in a plastic-like bag. This bag is implanted beneath the surface of the breast. The look and feel is more natural and normal, the chance of infection is minimized, and the cancer risk is eliminated.

Silicone works well when injected under scarred skin, but it is not permitted for this purpose, largely because of the problems it caused in its early history.

Fibrin, on the other hand, offers great promise as a means of "normalizing" age-scarred skin.

Facial Rejuvenation From Another Angle

We have discussed the many approaches to looking young again.

Altering facial contours and wrinkles is continually going on here on the "face" of mother earth. A forest fire burns off the old trees and permits new growth. Wind erodes top soil for plains. The sun creates sandy deserts.

The old adage "an ounce of prevention is worth a pound of cure" seems especially appropriate to this subject.

It is too late to talk about prevention to the person who is already "faced" with the mark of old age. It is to this person that this chapter has been dedicated.

But it is not too late to talk about prevention of aging marks to many others. Here is where the greatest changes take place.

I wish there were a way to show a picture of a person who did not take care of his skin to prevent aging, and then a picture of how that same person would look if he had taken even a modicum of care through the years. The contrast would be even more dramatic.

Facial *juvenation* is much more successful than facial *rejuvenation*. An ounce of sun protection, freedom from stress, and daily skin care are worth a pound of dermabrasion or plastic surgery.

In China, the old system of medical practice was to pay the doctor while you were healthy, not when you got sick. It was his job to keep you healthy. If he failed, your payments to him stopped until he restored your good health.

Unfortunately, we dermatologists seldom get to advise people with healthy skin to keep it young and healthy looking. We get to see people only as patients—when they already have a skin problem.

This book satisfies a great yearning on my part to get this "stay young story" across before skin gets old. Preventive medicine may one day be part of the American system. Preventive skin care has been emphasized throughout this book.

I close this chapter with an appeal similar to the appeal I made to you in the first chapter of this book. Be a skin vigilante. Add a new wrinkle to your skin awareness. Expand your duties as a skin vigilante to include the awareness of the subtle signs of aging in your skin: the folds, lines, and wrinkles. Analyze the probable cause of skin problems, with special attention to sun and stress—the two major physical and emotional causes of aging. Don't wait. Do what needs to be done right now to reduce the cause and alleviate the effect of skin disorders.

Create your own fountain of youth.

Home Care of Hair and Nails

What are hair and nails doing together in a chapter? They are both extensions of your skin. Your skin grows hair. Your skin grows fingernails and toenails. If you are not interested in strong, healthy fingernails and a full head of lustrous hair, there is no need to read this chapter. You may skip it. The rest of you, follow me.

The same elements of our environment that affect the skin also affect the hair and nails—sun, air, stress, vitamins, medications, viruses, germs, fungi, and poisons.

How to protect against these hazards and maintain attractive hair and nails with simple home care will be our main thrust. But we will also review when it may be necessary to seek the aid of a professional skin care specialist.

We will start with hair. Next to facial skin, the hair is of prime importance to acceptance socially and sexually. Healthy hair, properly managed, is as important to being in style as is the dress you wear or the cut of your suit.

Yet we often mistreat this important asset, either from ignorance or apathy. In the face of the abuse our hair receives, it is remarkable that it holds up as well as it does. Hair is a unique structural member of the skin we live in. The tensible strength of hair is so high, that if the fibers our clothes are made of were as strong, they would hardly ever show wear and tear.

Women are concerned with not only the desirable growth of a lustrous head of hair, but also with the undesirable growth of hair elsewhere on the body.

Hair control begins with the hair follicles. The follicles are the equivalent of the roots of your "crop," and there are said to be about one hundred thousand of these on the average female; more on the male.

People with straight hair want curly hair. People with curly hair want straight hair. Permanent waving solutions change the chemical bonds of the hair protein and permit you to change the natural characteristics of the hair. Once your hair is curled or straightened, another chemical fixes it that way. Hair stays straight or curly for weeks or months, but as new hair grows in, it returns to its original pattern.

Normal hair grows in cycles. We hae been able to identify three of these cycles. First, anagen (or growing cycle) lasts from three to seven years. Second, catagen (or regression cycle) lasts two weeks. Third, telogen (or resting cycle) lasts about three months. Your hair went through these three cycles in your childhood, and is still going through these cycles in adulthood. When these cycles are completed, so is the hair. New hair takes the place of old hair.

However, one hair does not keep in step with all of the other hairs. Each hair is in a different stage of growth. When you comb or brush your hair and hair comes out, that is resting hair. You are not necessarily "losing" hair. Its time has come. The old hair makes way for the new hair.

When you brush or comb hair that is in the growing cycle, you cannot pull it out. It is too firm, too strong. The average person loses one hundred hairs a day.

"Doctor, look at this! What can be wrong?" The patient shows me a ball of hair she has removed from her hairbrush.

'Have you looked in your vacuum cleaner? You'll find even more there," I reply. It is normal to lose a "wad" of hair. It is actually happening to you every day.

The Key to Healthy Hair

A healthy person has healthy hair. Show me hair that is less than healthy, and I'll show you a person with health problems.

When you take care of your general level of good health, you are taking care of your hair. Most treatments aimed at the health of the hair rather than at the health of the person do not work. For instance, if you take a vitamin because you have heard that this vitamin helps your hair, you are not going to get the results you expect. In fact, too much vitamin A can actually cause hair loss!

On the other hand, if your vitality is low because your diet does not include enough vitamins, anything you do to counteract that vitamin deficiency will definitely help your hair.

The same is true of gelatin as of vitamins. A large manufacturer of gelatin has claimed for its product hair and nail benefits. This manufacturer has made some studies that I consider "lukewarm," which purport to show that hair and nails grow faster and/or stronger when gelatin is taken by mouth. Most dermatologist feel that only a person who is not getting enough protein in his diet would be likely to find such a benefit from gelatin. Even then, this protein-deficient individual would probably have to eat twenty or thirty packets of gelatin a day to be able to attain observable improvements!

One common myth is that massaging the scalp helps to produce healthy hair. The truth is that massaging serves no useful purpose in building healthy hair.

Fiction: massaging the scalp improves circulation in the scalp and brings more blood supply to the hair follicles.

Fact: Your hair is getting its share of blood supply—massaging only pulls out hairs that are in the resting stage.

Since your hair is an extension of your skin, what harms your skin harms your hair.

To do your hair a service, avoid exposing your head excessively to skin enemy number one—the sun. The sun dries out your hair.

There are other "excesses" to which hair is commonly subjected. Too much heat, as from hair dryers, is one of these excesses. Overteasing hair can be an excess. Too much chlorine can be harmful to fragile hair. But unless the chlorine is used in quantities that exceed required limits, or unless you swim for long periods in pool water, chlorine will probably not have adverse effects on normal hair.

Assuming that you are taking as good care of your hair as you are of your skin, then the key to healthy hair is a healthy you.

Your total health is the key to a healthy head of hair, but a key without a "door" to use it on is not of much help. Later in this "visit" with you, I will discuss some of the doors available to you to advance your health all the way to the top of your hair.

Meanwhile, the quantity of hair can be a far more important problem to men and women than its quality.

How to Get Rid of Unwanted Hair

Usually, women are concerned with too much hair, men with too little. Hair quantity has genetic roots. For instance, Mediterranean women have more hair than women from northern Europe. The balance of male hormones when disturbed can accelerate the growth of unwanted hair. A sudden growth of unwanted hair can take place because a tumor is producing male hormones.

Similarly, hormones prescribed by a doctor can result in unwanted hair. Incidentally, the birth control pill usually does not do this. Oral contraceptives can actually cause hair loss.

Too much unwanted hair can be a serious cosmetic problem for women. There are several ways to handle this problem.

You can bleach unwanted dark hair on legs or arms to make it less conspicuous. The same is true of unwanted hair on the lip, the chin, or around the nipples. Black hair can be "unsightly" on a woman, whereas that same hair, if blonde, is acceptable.

Bleaching is not only simple to do, it is more emotionally acceptable to most women than the other common method of hair removal—shaving.

Most women—even those who still readily shave their legs and armpits—will cringe at the idea of shaving their faces. Shaving is like an instant sex change.

There are many good over-the-counter preparations for hair-lightening. Peroxide is the common constituent of these preparations. As long as you follow the instructions and do not leave the bleach on too long, there is no burning or adverse effect from these peroxide products. Peroxide bleaches are perfectly safe.

Bleaching is a continuous process. As the hair grows out in a few weeks, the procedure needs to be repeated. But then again, so does shaving.

Society accepts shaving by women on the legs and under the arms. Any kind of razor is fine—safety or electric, it really makes little difference.

Misconception: Shaving makes hair grow faster. This is simply not so. What happens is that the hair is a little coarser after shaving, because the base of the hair is thicker. It seems as though the hair is growing faster, but it is just sturdier.

Hair extraction is preferred by many women because it is a one-time process—at least for those hairs. Hair extraction is known as epilation. There are home epilation devices. Perma-Tweez is one. Perma-Tweez is an electric device, easy to use, but in my opinion not all that effective; yet many people like it. It is a battery operated device in the twenty-five dollar price range. Perma-Tweez has a fine electric needle.

To use Perma-Tweez, you insert the needle into the hair opening. The needle then dislodges the hair by heat-chemical reaction. It is a time-consuming procedure. Many persons have difficulty in seeing the hair opening, and in inserting the needle properly. Perma-Tweez has a safety device that cuts off the current if you go in at the wrong angle and miss the hair root, so it requires perseverance and patience.

Most of my patients have found it less "taxing" to hand the task of epilation over to a professional electrologist. The method is basically the same, but the equipment used is far more advanced and efficient. Still, electrologists can get rid of at best only about 80 percent of the unwanted hair in a given area, and possibly only half. The rest of the hairs have not been destroyed, and they do grow back. Those hairs that have been destroyed are gone forever.

A great deal of time is necessary for electrolysis. You lie on a table. The technician, using a magnifying glass, attacks hair after hair, by inserting the needle and turning on the current. The needle is hot, but not uncomfortably so.

A sex-transfer patient, male, came into my office to get rid of some of the now unwanted vestiges of his male existence. I referred him/her to an electrologist. It required some fifteen visits for this patient to accomplish the transformation, hair-wise.

Young women who enjoy the brief bikinis now in style come in for the removal of pelvic hair. I see these patients year after year, as bathing suit styles cover less and less of the body. Bikinis are keeping electrologists busy.

Another way to remove hair permanently is with wax. Hot wax is applied to the area of the skin covered by unwanted hair. The wax is permitted to dry and is then yanked off. With the wax comes the hair.

Wax epilation sounds barbaric, but it is not as painful as you would imagine. Wax epilation is quite popular in Europe, especially among women wishing to have leg hair removed permanently. Some people apply the wax themselves. However, many beauticians are trained in this procedure, and it is easier to let them handle it. Wax epilation needs to be redone several times in order to be permanent. It actually kills the hair by traumatizing it. And the trauma is not exclusively the hairs—your trauma can be diminished by keeping your thoughts very busy on other matters—like how attractive you will be when it is over.

The Causes of Hair Loss

Hair loss is largely a male problem, and is primarily due to genetic factors. Bald father begets bald son, and/or grandson. If a woman has a baldness problem, it is also likely to be genetic. As the woman gets older, the genetic factor takes over. Hormone changes take place which cause the loss of hair, for instance, on the top of the head, where indeed the same loss has occurred generations ago with the grandfather or grandmother.

Another common cause of hair loss is traction alopecia (hair loss). Traction alopecia is due to prolonged tension on the hair, for instance, due to a tight ponytail. This tension produces an inflammation that prevents normal growth of the hair, and if continued, the hair's demise. Once a ponytail hairdo is discontinued, any small bald spots it has produced will be largely covered by new hair, but the head will never be quite the same.

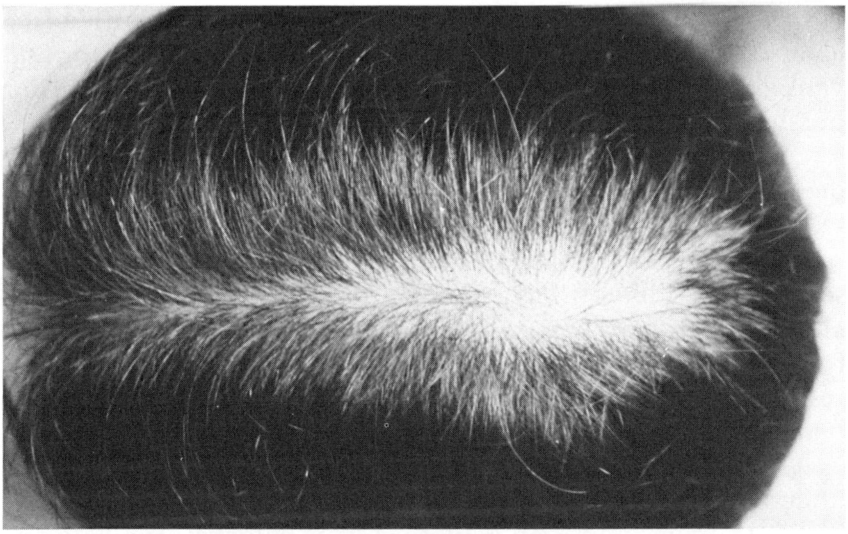

Hair loss (alopecia) at location of part due to ponytail.

The ponytail produces most tension on the frontal hair, so that is where the hair loss usually begins. It may not be noticeable to start with—only a slightly higher forehead is observable. Older Oriental women have high foreheads because they used to wear their hair in ponytails. Fortunately, the ponytail is not as in style today in our own younger generation as it was in the 1950s—at least not the tight ponytail that causes the trouble. Whenever I see a ponytail in the office, I say "loosen it up!"

Hair loss can also be caused by a hair style where the part in the hair is always worn in the same place. Because of constant brushing in the same place, that particular area begins to thin out due to traction at that spot.

Whenever I see a woman whose hair is thinning out at the part, I have her move the part a bit over to one side for awhile, and then back a bit over to the other side. Traction alopecia sometimes means permanent hair loss, so it pays to take steps today to avoid tomorrow's penalty.

We traumatize the hair frequently through improper management, and such traumas, too, can cost us permanent hair loss.

The most frequent abuses of the hair are brushing too hard

with a stiff nylon brush, or combing too strenuously with a fine comb. You might just as well pour hot wax on your head, and yank off the hair that way! Yanking out hair with a comb or brush pulls out growing hair.

These abuses cause small bald spots and thinning out of hair over a period of time. If you find sudden large patches of hairless scalp, you are in a different "ballpark."

Widespread hair loss is usually due to an infection. The person affected probably has a temperature. The problem could be a kidney infection or pneumonia. When the body's immunological forces are being severely challenged, or when the body's resistance is sharply lowered, the hair stops growing, as if the body needs the nutrients for higher priority use.

This is temporary hair loss. Once the infection is brought under control and the body's resistance normalized, new hair begins to grow, and even if there is total baldness, the baldness will soon be covered by new hair growth.

The birth control pill has been known to cause hair loss in women. This can be quite deceptive, because it may not happen until the woman has been taking the pill for a few years. Then hair loss occurs insidiously and gradually, so that it often goes unnoticed for quite awhile. Even after use of the pill is stopped, the gradual hair loss can continue for years. Sometimes the hair will grow back, sometimes not.

Other causes of hair loss include:

- Some medications (some chemotherapy and X-rays)
- Diet deficiencies (like iron)
- Thyroid imbalance (hypo or hyper)
- Postnatal conditions
- Liver disease
- Internal tumors or surface cysts
- Crash diets
- Emotional factors
- Poisons (like lead poisoning or thallium, a rat poison)

Sudden stress can cause alopecia areata. This is a round bald spot in the scalp. A stewardess involved in a minor air mishap had three such patches of hair loss soon after the accident.

Alopecia areata is a temporary hair loss. When the stress is over, the hair grows back. In the case of the stewardess, it took just a few weeks before new hair was fast eclipsing the bald disks.

We do not know why stress causes these bald spots to occur in circular shapes. It might have something to do with the immunization mechanism, which takes over to protect the rest of the hair.

Severe prolonged stress can cause alopecia totalis—complete loss of hair on the head—or even alopecia universalis; you guessed it, complete loss of hair all over the body—pubic area, eyebrows, everywhere.

The longer this condition persists, the less the chance of the hair returning. Treatment for alopecia universalis is available. Cortisone injected into the skin or into the buttock stimulates the

Hair loss due to nerve problem (alopecia areata).

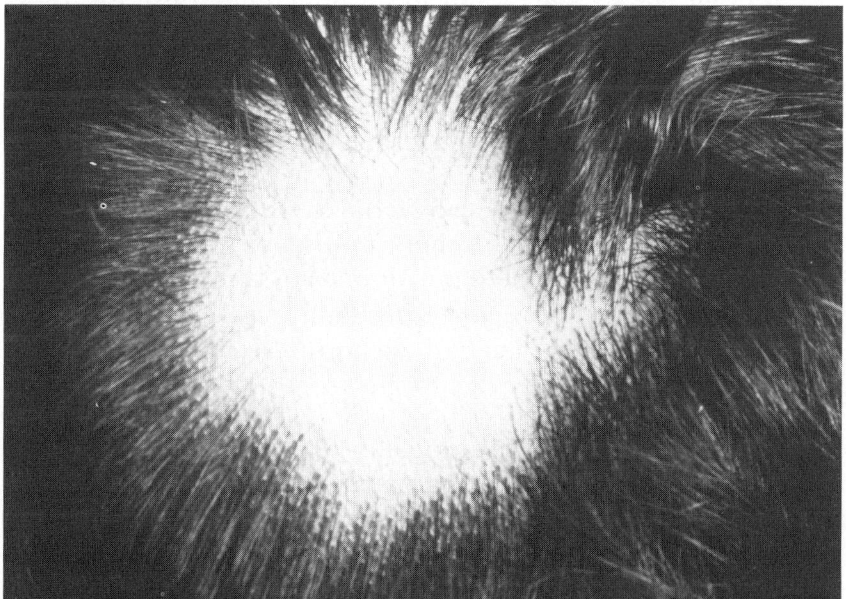

hair to regrow. It helps if the stress situation has been eased or eliminated.

This ability of the hair to regrow after sudden trauma holds for both physical and emotional trauma. Hair loss due to accidental intake of rat poision by a child is temporary. Once a disease that causes hair loss is cured, the hair usually grows back.

Scalp hair grows about one-half inch per month for the average person. This adds up to six inches a year. Hair can grow as long as four or five feet, but then it falls out as the growing cycle is ended, and the hair becomes resting hair. There are exceptions, but they are rare. Take a second look at the person with hair growing down to the ankles. This length is so rare, you may never see it again.

What You Can Do About Hair Loss

I have taken time to give you the many causes of hair loss, because the best thing that can be done for hair loss is to prevent it.

A great percentage of hair loss is only temporary. But there are bald men and bald women who will be bald no matter what they buy to stimulate hair growth, or what the ads say. In fact, dermatologists have noticed an increase of baldness among women, and this may soon be a visible sign of the equality of the sexes.

Can that "equality" indeed be the cause of female baldness? As women assume more and more roles that were formerly the exclusive prerogative of men, are more male hormones being produced? This is merely conjecture, but may one day be researched. While production of male hormones means a tendency to more hair on the body, it also means a tendency to a loss of hair on the head.

Many barbers and beauticians encourage treatments to overcome baldness. You have nothing to lose but money, but I personally doubt if you have much to gain, either. Most beauticians are sincere and conscientious. Still, they depend on selling their products and services. These products can, however, be beneficial for thin and fragile hair. For that reason alone, beauty parlor visits are well worth the expense.

There are also over-the-counter preparations for baldness, like Daragen. Daragen is a protein-type shampoo which actually thickens and strengthens the shaft of the hair.

When the causes for sudden loss of hair mentioned on the previous pages are relieved, removed, or ended, the hair will grow back. Occasionally, cortisone injections may be used to accelerate this restoration. This is so for alopecia areata—the round bald spots. The cortisone is injected with a needle and syringe or a "dermo-jet"—an air-injector gun similar to that used for polio or smallpox vaccinations. Hormone pills can also occasionally stop a hair loss, and even reverse it. Testosterone, a male hormone cream, can be applied to the scalp, where it stimulates the growth of hair. But one-quarter to one-half inch is the maximum growth producible by hormone treatments.

If your house has an unattractive feature, you can always grow ivy over it. if the skin you live in develops baldness, you can always consider wearing a hairpiece or wig.

"Will wigs interfere with the normal growth of my natural hair?" This is a question that I hear quite frequently. The concern seems to be that keeping air away from the scalp will make the normal hair suffer. The answer is: a wig causes no harm to natural hair.

Stress caused by the cosmetic liability of baldness can contribute to hair loss. If baldness is a source of stress for you, it is important that you cover the area with a hairpiece or wig, be you man or woman.

Surgery is now coming to the rescue of people with bald spots. Hair transplants are made from one part of the body to another. Plugs of hair are moved pretty much as sod might be transplanted to create a grassy area.

Usually, in males the hair plugs are taken from the sides or back of the scalp and moved to the top or front where the baldness is. The male back hair genetically due to the male hormone grows for longer periods. That is why back hair outlasts the front or top hair where baldness occurs.

Plastic surgeons can also transplant large strips of hair, instead of circular "punches." Moving large flaps means that more area can be covered with a single visit, but even so, this hair transplanting is a multi-visit procedure.

Another operation is now being performed, whereby a hairpiece is permanently fixed to the head. A tunnel is made in the skin, and the wig is sewn to the tunnel. The body does not reject the foreign hair, because the hairpiece is merely sewn over the scalp—and affixed with sutures.

Many men accept the genetic "heritage" of baldness. But when they become balder faster than their fathers or grandfathers, they hurry to their dermatologist crying "foul."

The answer is, of course, that they are treating their hair differently than their progenitors—or rather mistreating it differently. Emotional stress or physical stress may be the cause of premature hair loss. Can you imagine what fathers and grandfathers think of today's young and middle-aged men who blow, tease, and dye their hair?

Another solution to progressive baldness in successive generations could be the increase of mercury in the environment. Mercury is a toxin to hair growth. Mercury can affect hair growth even though it does not noticeably poison other parts of the body or cause illness. Mercury is in water, fish, and whatever eats those fish. It does not take large amounts of mercury to produce baldness; just trace amounts over extended periods can cause hair loss.

Support conservation measures to reduce pollution. The hair you save may be your own.

Your Nails' Worst Enemies

Nails grow at different rates. One person's nails can grow "at a fast clip." Another person's nails can appear to be hardly growing at all. You now know enough about the behavior of the skin you live in to explain this difference in rate of growth.

Of course, the rate of nail growth has to do with the person's level of good health. If your appetite, nutrition, and general health are good, your nails grow at a normal rate. The worst enemy of your nails can be your own body. Your body is the life-support system of your nails, so if it is not providing that support, the nails show it.

Healthy nails should be smooth, without ridges or grooves. They should be uniform in color and consistency, free of spots or discolorations.

Your beautician is skilled at masking nail defects. Besides adding color and gloss, cosmetic nail preparations can conceal the effects of trauma on your nails.

Your dermatologist, on the other hand, is interested in ending nail problems and defects.

Nail Problems and How to Prevent Them

The simple act of cutting your nails can be supportive or not to healthy nails. Nails grow faster at the sides near the edges of your fingers and toes than they grow at the center.

Hangnails occur because of this different rate of growth. If you have a hangnail, do not pull it off or bite it off: you can cause infection this way. Simply clip it off.

Toenails should be cut straight across rather than curved. Otherwise, when you walk, the sides tend to grow inward, and you develop what we term an ingrown toenail.

"Hangskin" is my own word to describe the skin that hangs flat from the hangnail cuticle area. You tend to pick hangskin off by pulling it back, which merely invites it to grow back. It is better to take a cuticle scissors and snip the hangskin off. The skin at the cuticle does not grow upward, as the rest of our skin does, but rather outward in the same direction as the nail. If cut evenly, the hangskin does not appear again.

Many women come into the dermatologist's office with cuticle infections. These women usually have horizontal ridges on their nails, where previous infections have made their mark. The usual cause of cuticle infections is overzealous beauty care.

Women or their beauticians can be too agressive in treating the cuticle. Nature has placed the cuticle where it is for a purpose. Cuticle is there to protect the nail. Pushing back the cuticle may yield a cosmetic advantage, but the price is the risk of nail damage and nail infection. Tampering with the cuticle opens the door to yeast, bacterial, and fungal infections. The half-moon you see means that the cuticle protects the growing part of the nail. The cuticle acts as a bandage for this living part of the nail.

If you must push back the cuticle, do it gently and moderately. There are jellies and other softening materials that you can put on the cuticle that lessen the chance of damage to this protective skin. I vote against pushing the cuticle back. If you do, at least you are now aware of the risks.

Some people are in occupations that traumatize their nails. A typist who spends most of the day hitting the keys is really spending most of the day hitting her nails. This can be like shock treatment to the nails. Typists should cut their nails shorter than they might like to, trading good-looking nails by dint of length for good-looking nails by dint of health.

People who dial the phone constantly should consider substituting a pencil or dialing device for their fingers.

Cutting your nails can be traumatic, too, especially if your nails are hard, and you have to exert a lot of force to accomplish the job. Nails are easier to cut after a bath, or if soaked before you cut them. Water quickly softens nails, and makes the cutting process less traumatic to them.

Soft nails that do not grow long enough are often the bane of the beauty-conscious woman. Probably tons of gelatin have been consumed by women who want to harden their nails. I don't know why these women are so susceptible to the advertisements for gelatin as a nail-hardener. Maybe their soft nails make them a "soft touch" for this kind of promotional information. Despite all the studies purporting to show a correlation between gelatin ingestion and nail hardness, I have yet to see convincing results.

One study back in 1950 reported that daily ingestion of gelatin corrected cracked and splitting fingernails. Since then a number of studies have been made, some later showing that the 1950 survey was in error, others corroborating the study but not accounting for the placebo, or "suggestion," effect.

Maybe the power of suggestion is the key to the success or failure of the gelatin treatment: if you believe that gelatin will harden your nails, the gelatin becomes like the white sugar pill often prescribed when a doctor cannot identify the cause of a symptom. You take the placebo, and lo and behold—the symptom disappears.

Sorry, but by what I have already told you, I have eliminated gelatin as a possible placebo to harden your nails. Once you know that a substance is a placebo its effect is lost. Would you like to try calf's liver?

A new system to produce long nails that requires the help of your beautician is called "Juliette Nails." Juliette nails is a

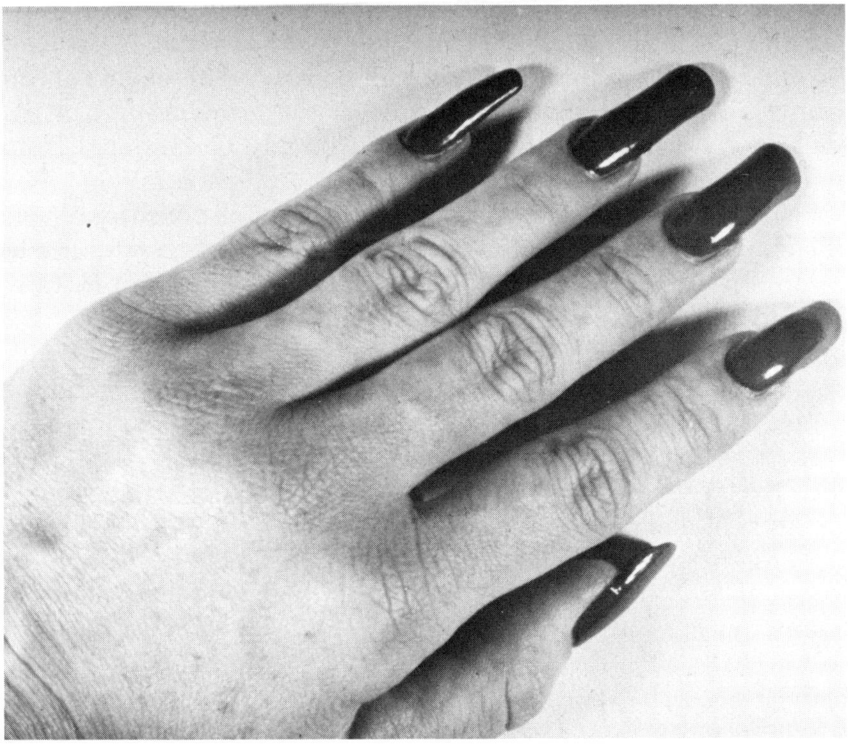

Juliette-treated nails.

method of using paper and glue to reinforce weak nails, permitting them to grow to an enviable length.

The beautician glues paper over the ends of the outer nails, covering about one-third of the nail. The paper is tucked underneath the tips of the nails, securely glued. Several coats of polish are then applied, giving the paper-covered nails a natural look.

The paper protects weak nails, permitting them to grow. You must lacquer the nails every second week. The paper does not strengthen the nails themselves, so the lacquering process must be repeated every two or three weeks, as the nails grow out.

Although stricly cosmetic and not therapeutic, the paper method seems preferable to other methods using harder substances sometimes called porcelain nails. These can break and harm the original nails.

Nail preparations, such as polish and polish remover, used cosmetically are quite safe. This was not always true. Years ago, formaldehyde was found in most nail polishes. This chemical can cause a contact dermatitis and irritate the growing part of the nail. Today, formaldehyde has been largely elmininated from nail polishes.

A chipped nail may not benefit from nail polish remover, the chip being equivalent to a small skin lesion. It is safer not to clean off all the polish with polish remover, which can irritate; instead, apply new polish over old.

Nail polish is more benign than polish remover. Polish remover acetone or acetone-like ingredients break the sulphide bonds that fuse the protein in the nail. A good rule to follow is: always go easy on polish remover. Prefer to put new polish over old. Excessive use of polish remover produces more fragile nails, as layers of nail peel off with layers of polish.

Again, the health of your nails depends on the health of your body. If you are lacking nutrients, the deficiency will show in many ways—low level of energy, low level of resistance,

Clubbing of nails due to pulmonary disease.

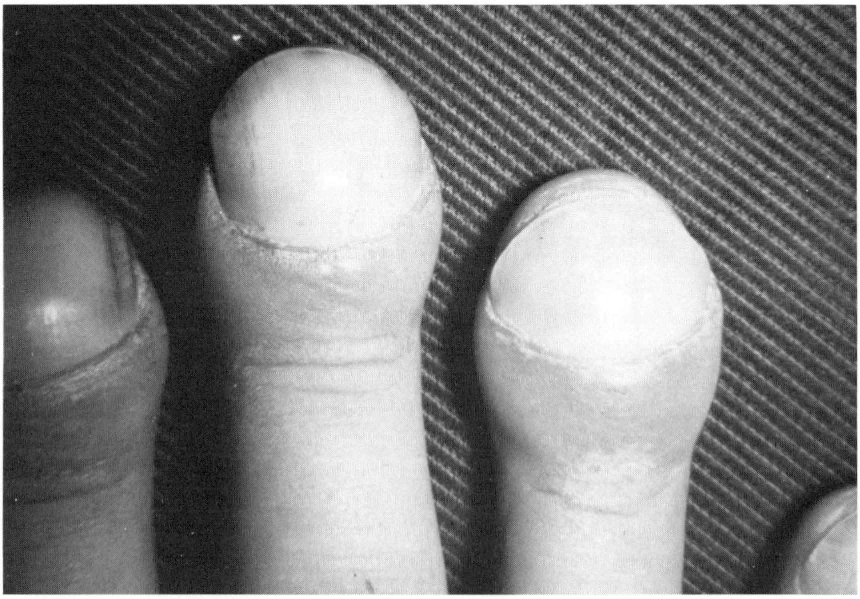

disorder, disease, and poor nails. Proper diet helps. If you are vitamin deficient, vitamins help.

If you have health problems and suspect that you might be nutrient or vitamin deficient, check with your doctor; or if you know you are neglecting yourself nutrition-wise, start eating correctly. If you suspect vitamin deficiency—and much of our food today is vitamin deficient—take a multi-vitamin. Then watch for an improvement.

Diseases of the Nails

Nails both reflect diseases in other parts of the body and are vulnerable to their own diseases. Nail abnormalities can signal such severe disorders as circulatory disease, endocrine imbalance, chronic poisoning, excessive radiation exposure, degenerative disease, and infection.

Nail changes in themselves seldom aid diagnosis of the problem, but some health problems make themselves seen in the nails first. So, if you detect a sudden change in nail color, or the appearance of spots, ridges or markings in the nails, it is wise to have your doctor check them. A telephone call to him might suffice.

Diseases that nails themselves can contract are not much different from diseases that affect the rest of your skin. Psoriasis causes pits and indentations in the nail plate—the hard part of the nail. When severe, these pits can be very deep, and destroy some of the nail. Eczema dermatitis, like contact dermatitis, can interfere with the growth of the nail plate, creating an irregular surface—ridgy, bumpy, jagged, and off-colored. Treating the eczema or psoriasis permits the nails to grow out looking normal once again. In severe cases, this is done by injecting cortisone under the cuticle. Benzoyl peroxide with cortisone cream is a newer and less painful treatment. A plastic cover or glove is worn over the ointment.

Fungus infections also occur on the nails of the hands or feet. Topical medications (placed on the nail) might work, but more effective is Griseofulvin—an oral pill that will be discussed in the next chapter.

Yeast infections of the nail are quite common, especially among bartenders, waitresses, and housewives. Identify a yeast infection as a round puffy area around the cuticle and sides of the nail. Press on the infection, and it will ooze pus-like liquid. Yeast infections can be painful. This is the same yeast that can grow and cause infections under the breast, in the vagina, and in other warm, moist places.

Diabetes predisposes a person to yeast infections of the nail or paronychia—meaning "around the nail." Anti-yeast preparations placed under the cuticle and around the nail help relieve paronychia. Gloves are *not* to be worn. In placing medication under the nail, do not poke it under: let the medication seep under the nail by capillary action.

Sometimes bacteria and yeast join together to infect nails. When bacteria are present, the swelling is greater, and there is more pus. Red streaks coming up the finger indicate blood poisoning. The medication for blood poisoning is antibiotics.

Older people with poor circulation often lose the hair on their legs. Nails show poor circulation also. They become off-color and ridged. Nails often crumble. Because Griseofulvin has a side effect of increasing or dilating the small blood vessels, it helps to restore circulation to the extremities, and has a therapeutic effect on crumbling nails.

If your dermatologist holds hands with you, Ms. or Mr. Patient, do not become alarmed. He has spotted many a case of emphysema this way, and maybe saved a life or two. He has spotted anemia, hyper and hypo-thyroid conditions, and other conditions that might have otherwise gone untreated. Your dermatologist can even spot clues to illnesses you have had in the past, like coronary or stroke. A tiny groove might be the giveaway, and the location of the groove enables your doctor to determine about how long ago the sudden illness happened. The growth—about one millimeter a week—provides the chart: it takes a fingernail six months to grow out.

Analysis of nails is being conducted in order to facilitate the diagnosis of mineral deficiencies like copper or magnesium deficiencies, cystic fibrosis, and other disorders.

A tip for older people and obese people who have trouble caring for their toenails because their nails become distended and troublesome. Use Keralyt, a salicylic acid jelly, to soften the

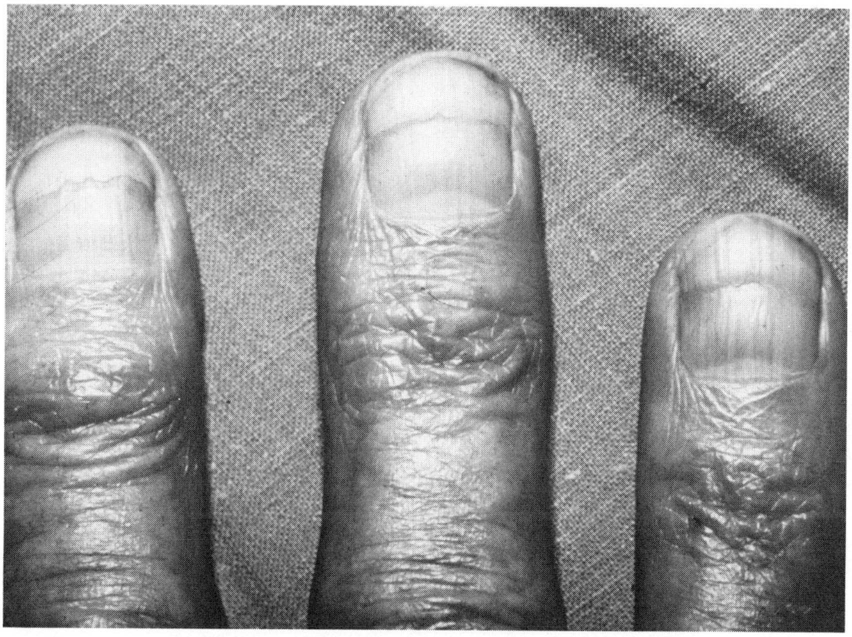

Grooves in nails show man had a heart attack about four months before.

nails. Keralyt is usually sold by prescription, and used with a plastic cover to help the softening process. After the application of Keralyt, a file permits the nail to be reshaped.

Hair and nails protect you—a special added bonus of the skin you live in. Nails were once man's only tools. Also his only weapons. Today, nails protect the ends of your active fingers and toes, while hair protects you from the elements. Nose and ear hair afford protection from foreign matter. Head hair protects like a hat.

Make this a mutual relationship. Protect your nails and hair!

Scabies, Fungi, and Tattoos

We want to touch as many bases as possible in alerting you to potential skin problems, so as to help you to prevent these problems as well as to treat them. Scabies, fungi, and tattoos are among the bases we have not yet touched.

One common denominator of scabies, fungi, and tattoo infections is their increasing prevalence. Scabies is currently approaching the stage of a worldwide epidemic. There is hardly a person alive who has never had some fungi problem; and the psychological need to adorn the skin, with the attendant risks and problems of such adornments, seems to be finding more and more expression, with not only tattooing on the increase but with other media, such as decals, being used as well.

The origin of these three subjects is quite different: scabies is caused by an animal—the mite; fungi is caused by plant growth; and tattoos are "self-inflicted."

Let's start by examining the little bug called the mite, which has millions of people scratching.

The Scourge of Scabies

Scabies has been around for a long time. Rumor has it that Napoleon's hand-inside-vest stance had the express purpose of scratching the scabies that he had on his chest. There is a good chance that this is true. Many a battle has been lost or won by the infestations acquired by soldiers.

Scabies has no preference for race, creed, sex, or color. It attacks rich and poor alike. I have treated top business executives and farm workers, office girls and society women.

Lice and scabies are not the same. Scabies is due to an even smaller creature than the parasitic louse that bites and sucks. The scabies-producing insect is called the mite. The mite does more than bite and suck: it burrows.

These mites that burrow into the skin can be picked up from a dog, cat, bird, or human. Usually, physical contact is required. So sexual relations are a common means of human-to-human spreading of scabies. When a dog has the scabies mite, the resulting condition is called mange.

Scabies starts off as a tiny water blister, maybe pinhead size. Then scabies forms a "trail," as it travels under the skin.

Scabies causes an irrepressible itching. The common sites for scabies to occur in humans are: in the fingerwebs, under the armpits, around the female nipples, in the navel, and in the groin.

Mother earth is burrowed by moles, which also leave trails. Human beings also attract burrowing mites, which choose particular sites on the body because they are warm and moist.

In the dermatologist's office, we could take a scraping of the scabies area and produce the mite under the microscope, but the condition is so typical that we just go ahead and treat it.

We treat scabies externally. The medication we use is called Kwell. Kwell, a milky liquid, comes in both a shampoo for the hair and a lotion for the rest of the body. Kwell is obtainable by prescription only. There are other, over-the-counter preparations that are just as effective as Kwell. One such medication is sulphur. Sulphur, which comes in a Vaseline base, is safe, and has been around a long while.

Kwell is a liquid lotion. You apply it with your fingers all over the body. It works the first time around, but the reason I recommend a second or third treatment is that you can miss parts of your body. Cover all the skin except in the eyes, ears, nose, mouth, and opening of the penis or vagina. Take a bath before applying the lotion. Change your clothing after the treatment.

You put Kwell on the entire body—not just where the itch

is. Keep the Kwell on for twenty-four hours, then wash it off. Kwell is not as sticky and messy as some of the other preparations. Patients appreciate this cosmetic advantage.

A teenage girl came into my office. She seemed embarrassed, and did not want to tell the nurse about her trouble. As she gave the usual history to the nurse, she kept scratching around her chest. When I saw her in the examination room, she was still scratching.

I looked at the girl's fingers. Between her fingers she had little water blisters. "Do you have itching under your armpits?" I asked her. "Yes," she replied, "How did you know that?" I continued to question her. "And around the belly button?" She nodded. "Groin?" Another nod. By this time she was totally confounded, because I seemed to know her intimate secrets in such detail. "And, of course, around your nipples." It did not take a Sherlock Holmes there, as this is where she was scratching constantly. "Scabies," I informed her.

The teenager admitted that her boyfriend had the "itch," too. I told her about the mite that gets under the skin, how it spreads, and how, if not treated, it can produce a general nerve rash over the entire body called neurodermatitis. "Your scabies can be treated effectively with this preparation," I said, showing her the Kwell. "But if your boyfriend lets his progress, he may need steroids—cortisone injections or pills, and anti-histamines." She promised that she would have the boyfriend come in for treatment.

Scabies has created an image that invokes frustration and disgust. Tell a patient that he has a mite called scabies that is living and multiplying under the skin, and he gets emotionally upset. Some patients start scratching everywhere the scabies isn't. Tell a student nurse that a patient has scabies, and the nurse starts scratching. One soldier who announces that he has scabies can get an entire army scratching. Scabies is not only a real physical itch, but it is an emotional "itch," too.

When one member of a family has scabies, every member of the family should be treated. One treatment of Kwell is usually enough, but it may be repeated once a week for three weeks, or three consecutive nights.

The clothing that is worn and the sheets and pillow cases slept on during this three-day period should be washed daily. You do not have to boil your clothing. Scabies is not a germ that needs to be sterilized in this way. The mite is removed from the clothing quite effectively by the washing process. Nor do you need to spray or fumigate the house.

It would pay to check your cat or dog for signs of bald spots—a symptom of the presence of scabies mites.

"I can't have scabies, Doc," insisted a bank vice president when I told him the nature of his itch. "I'm clean. I take a bath twice a day either at home, the gym, or the spa."

I then explained to him that scabies is not a result of uncleanliness or lack of personal hygiene. Scabies is a fact of life.

One man who came to see me with bumps on his skin all over his body explained that he had been itching for nearly two years, and thought it was emotional. When psychiatric treatment did not help, he went to a dermatologist, who recognized the scabies and treated it. But the doctor had not treated the man for the nerve rash that is a by-product of prolonged, untreated scabies. The patient was still sleepless, and more depressed than ever. A sleeping pill, a tranquilizer, and cortisone injections over a period of a week ended the sleepless suffering this man had experienced for two years, and he was able to enjoy life again.

There is a type of scabies known as Norwegian scabies, a name that sounds degrading to the Norwegian people, but probably has nothing at all to do with Norway. Norwegian scabies is very persistent. It seems to have a way of surviving, especially among older or debilitated people. Norwegian scabies seems to break down the skin, leaving wart-like formations. But Norwegian scabies is a rare condition.

Ordinary scabies is far from rare. The condition is widespread. Sometimes scabies arrives as an "epidemic." Recently, a nursing home called me, saying there was an emergency. I went down to the nursing home. All of the staff were scratching. I examined them. I found acne, psoriasis, sunburn, and warts, but no scabies. It seems that a doctor had discovered that one patient had scabies, and when the word got out, the whole staff started scratching. When I told the staff members that they did not have scabies, their itching stopped.

However, on similar calls I have had to tell the staff that they did have scabies, and that many of their patients had scabies. One such epidemic nearly closed a large nursing home.

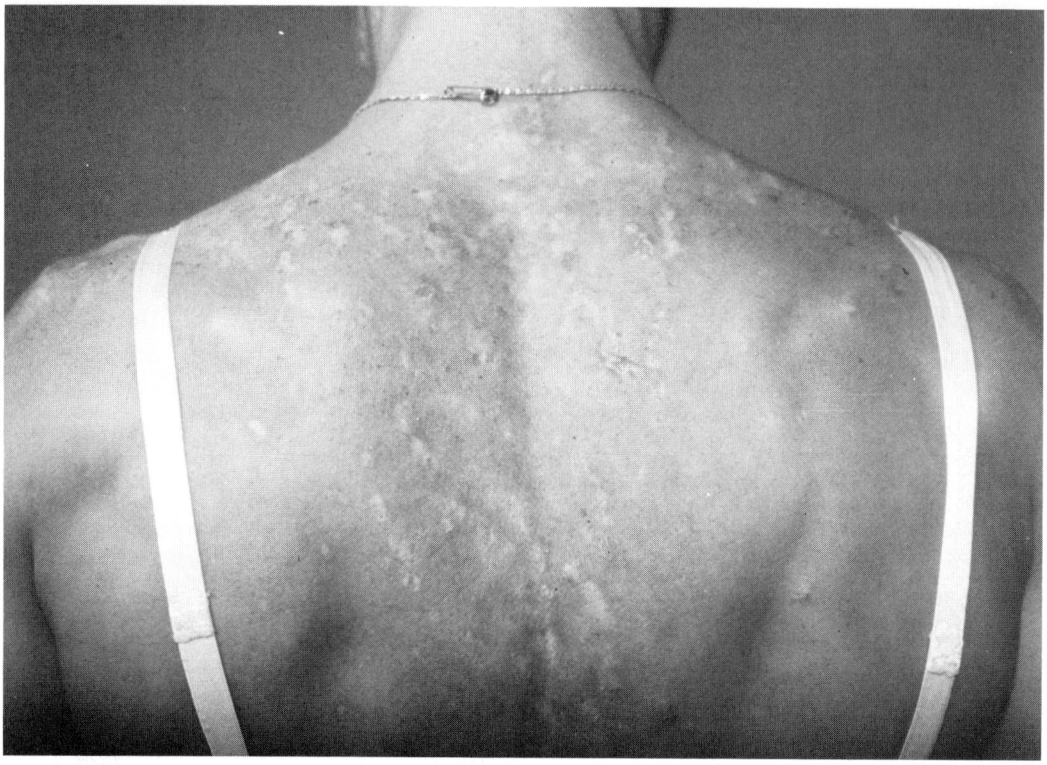

This woman, age fifty, had delusions of parasites. The marks are caused by the digging of her own fingernails.

Fast, thorough action ended the nightmare. This action included getting in an entomologist to track down the source of the mites. He found that when an exterminator had rid a storage room of termites, the mites that had been parasitic to these insects had to find another home, and spread quickly throughout the building to the staff and patients—through the air.

A woman got scabies. She insisted that she had no contact with other people or pets. We found that she slept by a window where many birds stayed, and the air was the mite "carrier."

The Louse and the Nit

Pediculosis is another infestation by an insect. Pediculosis is more commonly known as lice. The louse is large enough to see.

The insect looks like a tiny crab measuring about one or two millimeters. If you look carefully at the louse, you can see the crab-like legs extending out. The crab louse has pincers that hang onto the hair.

There are three main types of lice: body, head, and pubic lice. They do not burrow into the skin as do mites, but they are every bit as tenacious.

The pubic lice start off in the pubic area and tend to stay there. The head lice tend to stay in the scalp. The body lice claim the rest of the body for their domain.

The same treatment is used for lice as for scabies, and again, Kwell is preferred. One treatment usually suffices.

Lice can be spread by skin-to-skin contact. Lice do not live in the clothing. They need animate objects to inhabit. Nor are lice spread by birds or animals.

When I was a resident physician at New York Hospital, I had an interesting case. The patient was a married Orthodox Jewish woman. By tradition, such women are supposed to make themselves unattractive to men other than their husbands. One way of making themselves less attractive is to wear kerchiefs over their hair. Sometimes they wear wigs, or even shave their heads. This particular woman wore a kerchief. When I was asked to look at her, I removed the kerchief, and I saw what appeared to be dandruff. But the dandruff was moving!

Thousands and thousands of lice were making their home in this woman's hair, and had been for years. We gave her two shampoos with Kwell. She never felt so lightheaded.

The louse lays an egg called a nit. The nit is a cocoon-like organism that attaches itself quite firmly to a strand of hair. The cocoon does not protect the eggs or larvae from preparations like Kwell. So the nits die, but the only way to get rid of dead nits is with a fine comb.

You do not comb the hair in the usual way to remove nits. You need to comb from the ends of the hair toward the scalp. You hold the hair extended with one hand, as you comb inward toward the scalp with the other hand.

Lice and nits are spread at schools when children borrow each other's combs. Barbers keep their combs in alcohol to prevent communication of lice.

Lice become prevalent from time to time in one part of the

world or another. There was a time when people were "dusted" with DDT when they traveled from a lice-infested place to somewhere else, to prevent them from being carriers of lice. But the dusting was stopped when the toxic effect of this chemical was discovered.

Lice in the pubic area are commonly called "crabs."

A man came into my office and asked for treatment for pubic lice. He said he had seen them on his body and pulled them off, but still itched. After treatment with Kwell, he came back in a week, still itching. It seems he had forgotten to mention his girlfriend to me, or me to his girlfriend. This time, I gave him enough Kwell for two treatments—his and hers.

One girl came to see me complaining of a freckle on her thigh that itched. When I examined her, I found that the "freckle" was a large adult louse. Mature lice can become firmly attached to the hair. When the lice move, the itching is more severe. Since lice are more active at night, itching is worse at night for sufferers from lice and scabies.

I picked this large louse off the woman's thigh with a forceps, and put it under the microscope just to confirm that I saw what I thought I saw. I never show lice to the carriers, because the sight of the rather ugly creatures has a shattering effect on patients: they climb the walls. This monster I showed to my nurse after the patient left.

Fungi and Their Treatment

Tiny plants can also become parasitic on the skin you live in. Ringworm and athlete's foot are common examples of fungi, and both, incidentally, are misnomers.

Ringworm is not a worm. It is vegetation, a plant. Ringworm starts off as a little red spot, which grows peripherally. The reason the fungus then appears as a ring is because the body fights it, and the plant clears at the center. Sometimes you can see concentric rings where ringworm started, cleared, and started again.

Athlete's foot is another fungus, confined neither to athletes nor to the foot.

There are many kinds of fungi, some transmitted by people, some by dogs or cats.

If fungus grows in the groin area, it is called "jock itch," even if the host of the parasite is not a male.

When on the scalp, the fungus is usually called ringworm. Children get ringworm more often than do adults. In former times, entire schools would close down because of ringworm epidemics, but today treatment is too effective for the fungus to reach such proportions.

Adults can be more susceptible to ringworm when they are on immunosuppressive drugs for cancer, or on cortisone for arthritis, or have diabetes.

Also, people who perspire profusely are providing fertile ground for these plants to grow.

The home treatment for fungus is to keep it dry. If you can expose the fungus to the sun, this is effective. It also helps to put a

Superficial fungus infection.

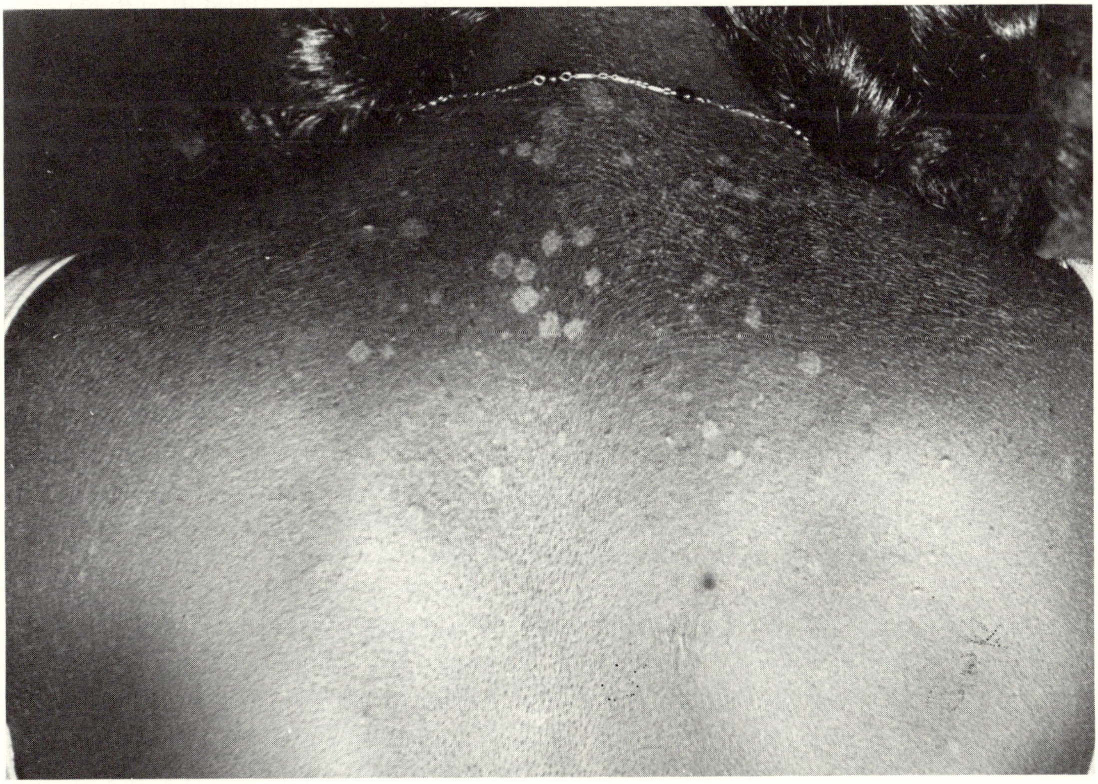

fan on and let the air blow on the armpits, groin, or wherever the fungus is. People who sit in cars a lot, like taxi drivers, get fungus of the groin and anus frequently. The condition can be alleviated by air conditioning of the cars, or by installing special foam-like cushions on the car seats.

You can see the fungus distinctly outlined as a red patch or as darker skin. You can see the plant disappear as exposure to sun or air cuts off the moisture it needs to survive.

Many over-the-counter preparations are excellent for treating fungi. The old Whitfield ointment is still around. It is a sulphur-salicylic acid preparation, most efficacious when put on the foot. Whitfield ointment dries and peels the skin. However, do not put this preparation on your testicles if you have jock itch: it burns intensely.

NP 27 is another good antifungal preparation, but again, not for the scrotum or genital area.

A newer antifungal ointment, which used to be sold only by prescription but is now sold over the counter, is Tinactin cream or solution. Tinactin actually kills the fungus, while the older creams derive their effectiveness from peeling off the skin. Tinactin is usable on the scrotum.

When fungus infections are widespread on certain parts of the body, such as hair and nails, it is best to treat them internally. Years ago, treatment of fungus on the nails consisted of removing the nails, because the fungus infection became so deep. A few years ago, we used to give X-ray treatment to the hair and scalp, hoping that if the hair was lost, it would return. Nothing else worked for treatment of fungus infections of the hairs and nails.

Now, we have a medicine taken internally called Griseofulvin. Griseofulvin is the generic name; there are also several trade names for the medicine. Griseofulvin gets into the blood stream and kills the fungus. It does not matter where the infection is—hair, nails, or widespread—one pill a day after meals kills the fungus in three weeks. Taking Griseofulvin after a meal helps absorb the medication into the blood.

Griseofulvin is quite safe, but it is a sun sensitizer. So you need to watch sun exposure while taking Griseofulvin but other contra-indications are quite mild and rare. (If patients are taking a blood anticoagulant, that dosage needs to be regulated.)

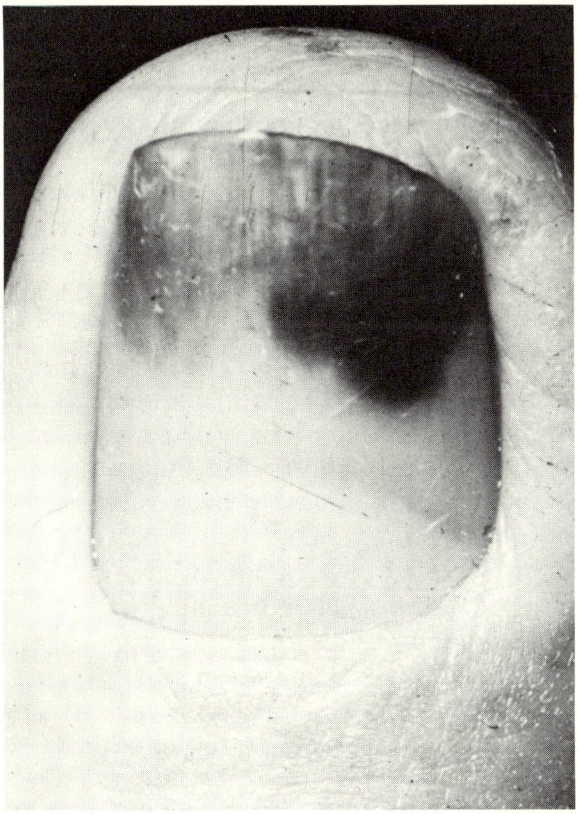

Fungus infection on fingernail.

Griseofulvin is quite reasonable in price, running (at this writing) about thirty-five cents a tablet.

I have seen patients who have had itching for twenty years from fungus stop scratching in just two or three days. The rash is still there, but the fungus is already beginning to be throttled. Griseofulvin works for all fungi, including what we call ringworm.

I mentioned that sun helps to kill fungi. Any dry heat helps. Ultra-violet lamps help, but not the heat lamps. The heat lamps cause sweating; the fungi can stand heat, and they enjoy moisture.

Sun does not kill all types of fungi. One Samoan fisherman had fungus rashes all over his body. Being in the sun all day was not helping him to get rid of the infection. He had to take Griseofulvin to end this condition.

Fungus infections of the scalp usually require the internal

approach. The Griseofulvin pill takes longer to work, and usually requires a period of six to eight weeks.

Yeast is another type of fungus. When you scrape the skin to take a culture or sample of yeast, it looks slimy like mucous, not fluffy like other fungi.

Yeast also thrives in warm, moist areas, such as under the breast, in armpits, and around the groin.

You can tell the difference between yeast and other fungi. While most fungi are sharply defined, the yeast produces satellite areas beyond the main infection. If you have a red groin and a few red patches beyond it, this is probably a yeast fungus.

There is a high incidence of relationship between yeast infections and diabetes.

Griseofulvin does not work for yeast infections. To treat yeast, we use external medications. They are all prescription. One is Vioform. Nilstat is another. Vioform and Nilstat kill the yeast.

Women commonly get yeast infections of the vagina. The yeast of fungal vaginitis is the same fungus as that in other yeast infections. Fungal vaginitis is treated with a cream, twice a day.

Yeast or fungus infections are not bandaged after treatment. We want the air to get to the infected area. Bandages increase the temperature and moisture of the skin.

People sometimes think they have fungus inside the ear. This is not likely to be so. The itching they feel usually comes from acne. This is treated with anti-dandruff shampoo, and clears up.

Remember, ointments and salves that are greasy worsen rather than improve fungus conditions. Rather than use such preparations, go to your pharmacist and tell him your problem. Your pharmacist is your friend. He can give valuable assistance with fungus problems, recommending over-the-counter preparations that are appropriate.

If you use a preparation for athlete's foot or other fungus and the itching increases, stop using the substance. You may be allergic to that preparation.

Also, do not use one preparation right after another. You are asking for contact dermatitis or other trouble. Pause in between different treatments. Let sun and air have a crack at the fungus before trying a new preparation. It may turn out that you won't need the medication.

For athlete's foot, put a cork between your toes while watching TV. Cotton is not a good substitute for the cork, because cotton does not cause a physical separation between the toes. Alcohol kills some fungi, but it burns the skin where the fungus is growing. The same is true of iodine. Betadine is better. Betadine is the preparation that was sent with the astronauts to the moon, and also used on reentry to sterilize the capsule and astronauts. It is sold over the counter, and does not stain.

Again, remember your pharmacist. He is a "partner in medicine" to your physician. Also, if in doubt, phone your doctor. Most doctors welcome phone calls. I tell my patients to call me any time of the day or night. Usually they respect my privacy and do not abuse the privilege. Your physician's experienced nurse can also save you time and inconvenience.

Fungus infection on toenail.

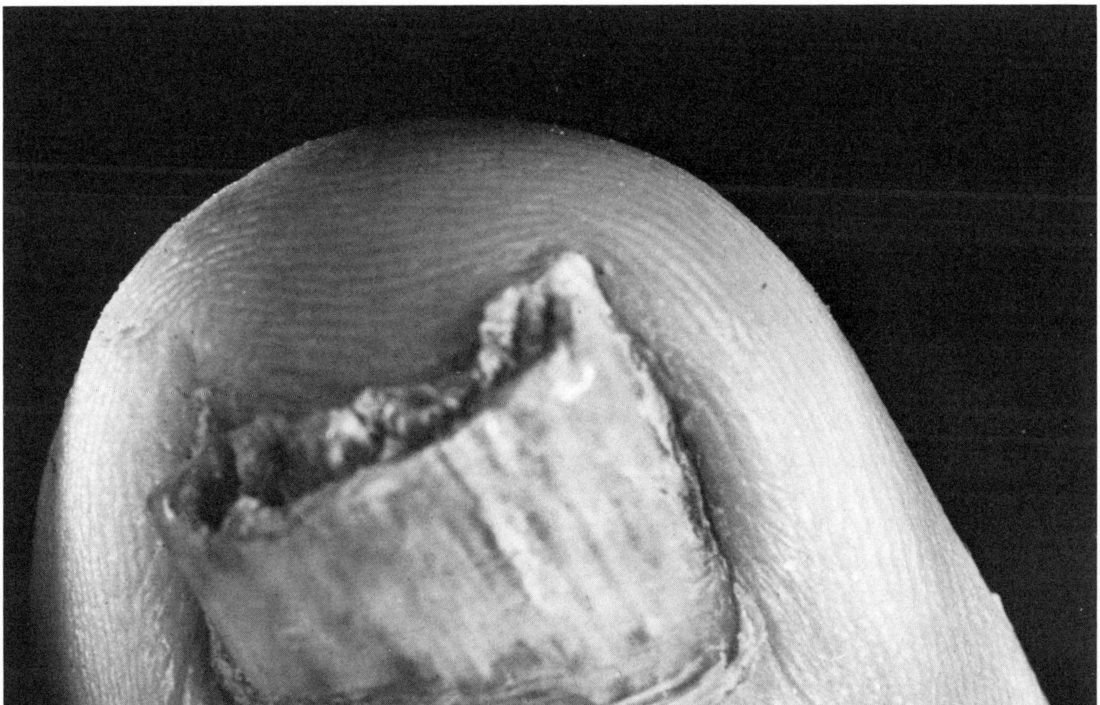

Pros and Cons of Tattooing

The scene is the heart of Los Angeles. A well-dressed secretary, age twenty-one, is about to have a butterfly tattooed on her left breast. The tattoo artist turns on a machine. The machine makes a buzzing, grinding sound.

"It won't hurt," says the artist, but the girl flinches as the needle touches the tender white skin of her breast.

Five minutes a later, a black outline has been etched on her now red and irritated skin. Next come the colors, deposited by tiny pools of red, green, and yellow dye. What does not sink in is wiped off and scraped, and the process is repeated several times.

The tattooing machine has several needles that vibrate lightning-fast, making one to three thousand punctures a minute in the skin about one-sixty-fourth of an inch deep.

Tattooing is on the rise. The last few years have seen women frequenting tattoo parlors in increasing numbers; men, also. Women favor a rose on the leg, "chocolate" and "vanilla" on the breasts, a butterfly on the stomach, an astrology sign on the thigh, a sunburst on the shoulder, a red devil on the buttocks and a lover's name wherever the spirit moves her.

Men still favor the eagle and snake in battle on the back, the skull and cross bones on biceps, and "Mother" blazoned across the chest.

People have been adorning the skin for millennia. According to the Tattoo Museum and Hall of Fame in San Francisco, tattooing began in the Stone Age some fourteen thousand years ago. Historical evidence begins with Egyptian mummies preserved over four thousand years.

Today, tattoo artists are in every large city, with Hong Kong, Honolulu, Tokyo, and Bangkok acquiring for themselves reputations as the tattoo capitals of the world.

A tattoo may take only twenty minutes to complete. But the discomfort tattooing entails may not end there. In fact, it may only be beginning.

I have nothing against the adorning of the skin, be it by war paint, decals, or tattoos. However, my dedication to the health of the skin you live in mandates that I warn you of certain skin hazards implicit in tattooing.

The problem is being compounded by the advent of

cosmetic tattooing. This is the use of tattoos to rid the skin of birthmarks, scars, or even old tattoos. A popular female television star is said to have a rose and butterfly tattoo to hide the discoloration on her derrière. People whose eyebrows have been burned or plucked off sometimes tattoo simulated eyebrows in their places. There is even vanity tattooing going on, like changing the arch of the eyebrow.

Certain pigments used in tattooing can give you trouble. Let me explain.

Sunlight and Your Tattoo

For decades, sailors with tattoos have developed itching eczema. Also, they have developed warty nodules on the red parts of their tattoos. This was suspected to be an allergic reaction to the red dye made from cinnabar (mercuric sulfide), and therefore a type of hypersensitivity to mercury. However, the cause and effect relationship between the dye and the allergy was never fully established, and the tattooed people continued to scratch, some developing sarcoid-like granulomas, serious lesions of the skin that could easily lead to infection, and possibly internal complications.

Between 1965 and 1967, I had the opportunity to study some fifteen cases of military personnel who had allergic reactions on the red tattoo sites. None of the fifteen were exposed to mercury, but all had considerable exposure to the sun. Previously, it had been noted in a Swedish study that a photo-allergic reaction occurred in yellow tattoo sites when tattooed men left Sweden and went to tropical areas.

After some allergy sleuthing using patch tests and biopsies, I was able to identify the culprit as cadmium sulfide, an ingredient common to both yellow and red tattoo pigment. Cadmium sulfide is a photosensitive chemical, and when exposed to sunlight, was causing the persistent problem.

My findings were later published in the *Annals of Internal Medicine* with the following comment by the editor, J. Russell Elkinton, M.D.: "Goldstein has solved the case of the itching tattoo with a deftness that would do honor to the Master Sleuth of Baker Street, himself a student and connoisseur of tattoos."

My advice to future tattoo subjects: avoid red and yellow dyes that contain cadmium sulfide. If you do have a tattoo, and if it must be exposed to the sun, use a sunscreen preparation prior to each exposure.

Psychological Aspects of Tattoo

Just as your inner states of anxiety and stress can cause psoriasis, acne, and other skin "markings," so can the markings we call tattoos have psychological causes.

We seek the tattoo because of certain emotional needs. Understanding and handling this fact might lessen the need for tattooing our skin.

Recently, I collaborated in a study of fifty psychiatric patients, all of whom had multiple tattoos. One tattoo is not indicative of emotional problems. It can be the result of a spur of the moment "lark." A number of tattoos can be indicative of an emotional problem, which is not solved by the tattoos any more than stress is relieved by psoriasis. If tattoos relieved emotional problems, maybe they would be worth the photosensitivity symptoms, the itching, the sarcoid-like granulomas, the skin tumors, and the risk of hepatitis from unclean needles. In 1961, New York City bannned tattoo artists after 13 of 243 cases of serum hepatitis were traced to tattooing.

In the study on which I collaborated, we compared the fifty tattooed psychiatric patients with fifty who were not tattooed. The evidence pointed to multiple tattoos scattered over the body as indicative of personality problems, while a large, single tattoo frequently pointed to schizophrenia.

The association of excessive tattooing with potentially antisocial behavior has emerged in actual crime cases. When identified on nationwide broadcasts, the tattoo of mass murderer Richard Speck, including the words "Born to Raise Hell," helped to locate the criminal.

Truman Capote, in his nonfiction book, *In Cold Blood*, described in great detail two jailed killers' tattoos. Dick Hickok had a grinning blue cat on his right hand, a blue rose on one shoulder, a human skull caught in the jaws of a dragon along with a pitchfork-brandishing gremlin on his torso, and other tattoos. Perry Smith had fewer tattoos, but his were more elaborate, like a snarling, red-fanged tiger on his left biceps, with a snake coiled around a dagger slithering down his arm. Elsewhere on Smith's body were skulls, flowers, and tombstones.

Removing Tattoos

My personal feeling about tattoos is: if you want a tattoo, have it done. If you do not want one, rejoice.

An attractive woman in her late twenties came into my office to ask my advice about getting a tattoo. This woman was the wife of a prominent attorney. I reminded her that a tattoo was a permanent "decision"; that it could be removed only by skin dermabrasion or plastic surgery; and that, if it was red and exposed to the sun, the tattoo could result in itching and more serious skin problems.

Her tattoo was to be small, she assured me, below the bikini line, where only her husband could see it; but she insisted that it would have to be red. I assured her that if the tattoo were covered in the way she described, there should be no problem.

The attorney's wife left, and very likely now a red flower blooms on her white buttock. But she may be back to see me some day. She may want to have the tattoo removed.

There are many reasons for a change of heart, depending on the nature of the tattoo and where it is located.

It might be a great idea one night to tattoo "Susie" on the end of the penis, or "Mike" on the bosom, but later the tattoo can become a source of unending questions and embarrassment. A tattoo on the forehead is a similar disaster. Maybe it was a good idea at the time, but now the pictorial star, eye, or whatever practically precedes you wherever you go.

One woman who thought she was a goddess in her commune had had a star with wings attached to it tattooed on her forehead. Then she had come down to earth, and had to wear a kerchief over her head and forehead at all times.

A man with one tattoo on his arm is not likely to want the tattoo removed, but people with tattoos in more bizarre locations are usually candidates for ultimate removal.

There are three basic ways to remove the tattoos.

First, a tattoo can be excised. This means cutting the picture out, and bringing the edges of the adjacent skin together to cover the spot. If the tattoo is two or more inches wide, it might have to be excised in installments.

Excision can also use new skin that can be grafted in place of the tattooed area. The skin is usually removed from the buttock. However, it never matches the part of the body to which it is grafted. A plastic surgeon is not a magician. He cannot make incisions disappear entirely, or make buttock skin match chest skin. match chest skin.

A second method of tattoo removal is by abrasion. The tattoo can be scraped off. Tattoos can be pretty deep. So abrasion means scraping well down into the fatty or subcutaneous tissue. Often, you do not get rid of all of the tattoo, but only of most of it. The method of abrasion for tattoo removal is the same as the dermabrasion described for other skin conditions.

The forehead tattoo once was a good idea. Now a bandana covers it.

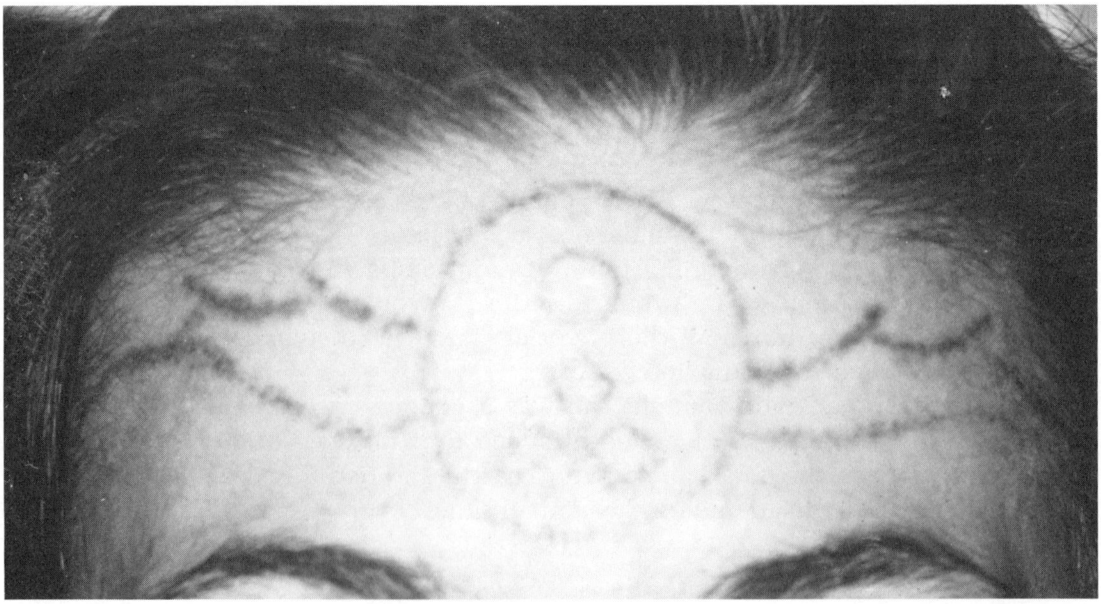

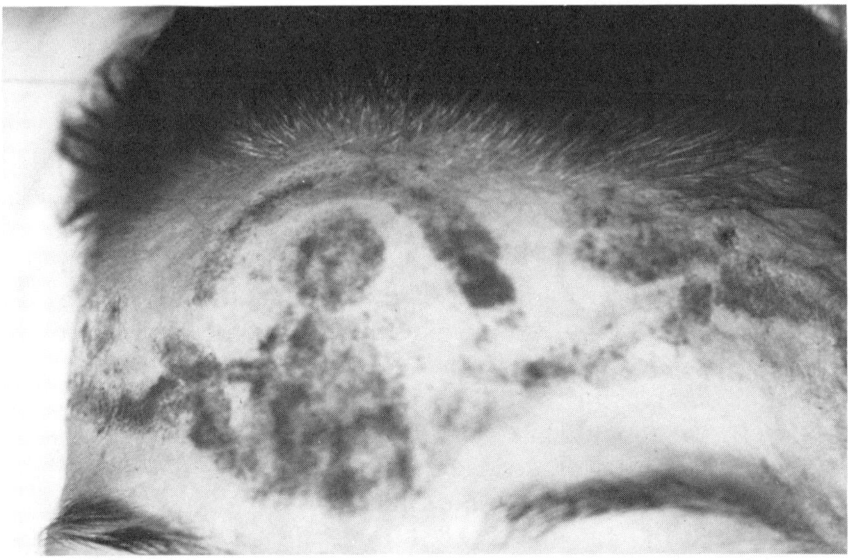

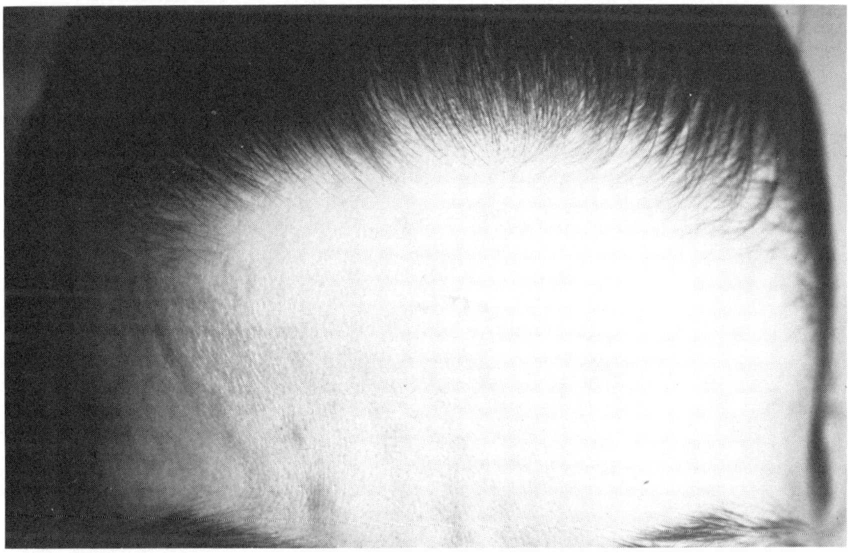

(Top) *Forehead tattoo minutes after scraping.*
(Bottom) *Forehead tattoo two months later.*

There is a "do-it-yourself kit" called salabrasion available at grocery stores. Salabrasion is actually kosher or coarse salt. You simply rub the tattoo with it, and although the treatment hurts, it does an effective scraping job.

A third method of tattoo removal is cryosurgery—freezing the tattoo off with liquid nitrogen. Cryosurgery is the most pain-free and the easiest method of tattoo removal, but again, you may not be able to get rid of all traces of pigment. If at the end of several treatments two or three weeks apart there is no dramatic removal, I stop using cryosurgery. At this point, I may recommend more tattooing: the use of the white pigment titanium dioxide over darker pigments. The new pigment makes the skin look closer to normal. Some plastic surgeons use the titanium dioxide approach.

The complexities of tattoo removal are such that you would do well to consider whether or not it is easier to seek psychological or psychiatric counseling, rather than wind up, as one patient I saw did, with multiple tattoos of "Sally," "Janice," "Mary," "Rita Hayworth," "Marlene Dietrich," and others. Such successive emotional attachments can often be better handled with a counselor's professional talent than a tattoo artist's.

Ten Commandments for Perfect Skin

As you now already know, my philosophy for skin beauty and attractiveness goes more than skin deep.

Women have found little on these pages about washing creams and cleansing creams, lipstick and mascara, hair frosting or dyeing.

Men have found little on these pages to guide them in the selection of shaving creams or shaving lotions.

There are hundreds of volumes on cosmetic skin care, and thousands of magazine pages on the subject are published every month.

"Cosmetic" is defined by the American Heritage Dictionary as a way of decorating the body that is "superficial rather than functional."

Which do you choose: a cosmetically decorated skin, or a functionally attractive skin?

Some functionally attractive skins can be strikingly beautiful, with no cosmetic help at all. Some functionally unattractive skins can never be made attractive, no matter what cosmetics are used.

How to achieve functionally attractive skin has been the thrust of my counsel to you. With functionally attractive skin, cosmetics can be used for finishing touches to the complexion, rather than as the foundation for skin beauty—a false foundation, which even the nearsighted and farsighted can see through.

Besides providing a foundation for genuine attractiveness, a healthy skin furnishes another interesting dividend. There is less chance that any particular soap, cream, or cosmetic will be irritating to a functionally sound skin than to a less than healthy skin.

Men who follow the basic guidelines for functionally healthy skin will find women attracted to them far more than men with unhealthy skin who use a scented after shave lotion with a French name. And their male colleagues will envy their virile and youthful look.

Women who follow the basic guidelines for functionally healthy skin will radiate femininity, and look years younger. Other women, not "in the know," will ask about your cosmetic secrets, and be amazed that you have none.

In this chapter, you will find summarized ten basic rules to follow for functionally healthy skin—skin with a natural attractiveness. Skin that is naturally alluring, naturally seductive, and naturally lovable. And such skin can also be cosmetically endowed with these qualities to a level of perfection worthy of even Hollywood's beauty-describing superlatives.

Emily Dickinson said, "Beauty is not caused. It is." As you follow the basic rules of this chapter, your beauty and attractiveness *is*.

"Beauty is the first present Nature gives to women, and the first it takes away," according to French writer George Brossin Méré. When you follow the functional rules for attractive skin, Nature postpones her "taking away" for decades.

"There is no cosmetic for beauty like happiness," said the Countess of Blessington. She could have been quoting her dermatologist, for certainly, finding the key to that happiness will be part of my guidance to you in this chapter—one of the ten basic "commandments" for perfect skin.

Let's begin.

The Basic Rule to Follow for Perfect Skin

In my considered and experienced opinion, the most important word in skin care is "moderation." The First Commandment of skin care is: be moderate in exposing your skin to the elements and to any kind of treatments.

It does not really matter to what you expose your skin, as long as exposure occurs in moderation. The skin has evolved over millenia through exposure to the elements, to plant and animal substances, and presently, to chemical detergents and other modern, synthesized preparations. The skin can take just about anything in its stride, in moderation.

A little sun is fine for your skin. A little cold cream is all right (if you don't have acne). A little heat, a little cold, a little soap are also desirable. Moderation is the key. The skin is strong. It rebounds. The "pH" of the skin adjusts itself, and other factors that are strained normalize if given the chance.

Excess of just about anything can cause wear and tear on your skin—even fresh outdoor air.

That ruddy outdoor look of the farmer may not be all that healthy. Analyze that look as a skin vigilante would, and you see irritation and aging.

I would be hard put to single out any factors that affect the skin that would be exceptions to this rule of moderation—except, perhaps, rest and peace of mind. As Longfellow said, "Joy and temperance and repose/ Slam the door on the doctor's nose."

Medicate a skin condition too much, and you can cause contact dermatitis; wash the skin too much, and you can rob it of its natural and needed oils. Stretch the skin too much, as in obesity or pregnancy, and you create stretch marks.

You cannot be moderately pregnant, and so stretch lines are a necessary "evil," more so for some women than for others, usually depending on genetic factors. Only plastic surgeons can undo the signs of immoderate stretching.

In other matters, you are in control. You can permit excess. You can be moderate. It does not matter "what" you use to treat your skin. What matters is "how much."

Choose moderation.

Know Your Skin's Worst Enemies

The most important thing to be moderate about is the very

thing that is in greatest abundance, and causes skin the greatest wear, tear, and damage—the sun.

We devoted a whole "visit" together to the discussion of the sun and the hazard it presents to your good looks and healthy skin. Knowledge about the effects of the sun on your skin and your vigilante attitude toward excessive exposure to strong sun can do more to prolong your youthful appearance than all the cosmetics ever invented.

You do not have to reread the chapter on sun to remind yourself of the effects of the sun. Just take a moment now to compare the skin on your face with the skin on your buttocks.

Commandment number two: protect your skin—with sunscreen preparations, if necessary—from excessive sun exposure.

The Third Commandment for healthy skin is to use soap and water—the right soap, the right water, and the right frequency. The skin needs to be washed periodically of environmental deposits.

Washing removes sweat, skin debris, sebum (which is an oily secretion), dust, grime, cosmetics, and whatever germs are attached to these substances.

Most soap is alkaline. alkali can irritate some skins. Normal skin is not harmed by most soaps. But abnormal skin may not be able to "rebound" from continued alkali. Where ordinary soap causes irritation, soap substitutes should be used.

Deodorant soap is a misnomer. Any soap deodorizes by cleaning. Soap marketed as a deodorant usually contains an antibacterial agent plus a perfume. Antibacterial soaps have the agent, but usually not the perfume. Medicated soaps should not be used as an everyday substitute for ordinary soap. Let your doctor advise you when to use medicated soap.

As a rule, there is less alkali in transparent soaps (sometimes called glycerin soaps) than in conventional toilet soap. One such soap is Neutragena. This is a very mild soap substitute, available in a bar for babies, for acne, and for dry skin.

Detergents are different from soaps in composition, but generally accomplish the same purpose. Soaps are manufactured from animal and vegetable oils, while detergents are synthesized from petroleum. Detergents "work" better when the water is hard or highly mineralized. Detergents leave less of a hard water scum or deposit than does soap. There are soap substitutes with less alkali in them than in soap. Some brand names of soap substitutes are Lindora, Lowilla, Aveeno, and Basis. The latter is superfatted for treating dry skin. Most come in cake form; Lindora is a liquid.

There are many skin care products that are sold for use in the bath. Some are neutral, others are not. Bath crystals that provide a fragrance are neutral. But bath salts, which add alkali, can be an unnecessary "load" for your skin.

Women with dry skin might alternate between soap and water and cleansing cream to clean the skin, but women with oily skin should use only soap and water.

Twice a day washing of the hands and face should suffice as a maximum; however, in cold weather once a day might be a preferable maximum for some people. Too much soap, too much scrubbing, or water too hot can make two of your skin's best friends (soap and water) into its worst enemies.

There's that First Commandment operating again: moderation.

Let's look at proper use of shaving and cosmetic preparations.

Most shaving and cosmetic preparations today are perfectly safe. Hypoallergenic is the word that describes them best. Hypoallergenic means less likely to cause trouble, but not necessarily trouble-free.

If you have a skin reaction to any product, stop using that product, and try another.

For instance, some lipsticks cause inflammation and irritation. If this happens to your lips, change lipsticks. If the condition persists, there may be a factor involved other than allergy to the lipstick.

Some perfumes contain a photosensitizer, and can cause brown spots when used on exposed areas. Some after shave lotions have been found to cause brown spots for the same reason.

Using someone else's eye makeup can cause you an irritation or infection, even if the owner suffered no such problem. High school girls who borrow each others' eye liners or mascara are encouraging the spreading of bacteria.

To cause as little trauma as possible to the skin when

shaving—man or woman—wet the beard or hair before starting. A little-known fact is that wetting the skin a moment before shaving is almost like no wetting at all. It is better to give the water time to work into the hair in order to soften the hair more effectively. You will get a better and a closer shave from this premoisturization. But also, you will be pulling and scraping the skin less—traumatizing it less, albeit the trauma of shaving is quite minor.

If you have a tendency to acne, be aware of oily preparations and avoid them.

Be aware of cosmetics that are photosensitizers. Know what you are putting on your skin. If an after shave lotion stings, that's what its astringent effect is supposed to do, but if the sting stays longer than the time needed to "wake you up," the lotion could be irritating your skin. Cheap products, made with coarser materials, tend to be more irritating to the skin.

So the Fourth Commandment for healthy skin is: know your cosmetics, and use them skillfully. Don't experiment with untried substances, like some plant juice that you think might be interesting to use. A large number of organic substances are poisonous to the skin. Before a cosmetic manufacturer uses such substances, many research tests are conducted on them.

Play it "Cool" Treating Your Skin

The Fifth Commandment for perfect skin is: "play it cool" when treating a burn or injury.

The moment that burn appears, or that cut or bruising blow occurs, your skin is already at work doing what needs to be done to repair the damage. We can help or hinder the action of the skin. Often, we get in its way.

The safest thing you can do to help your skin when burned or bruised is to apply cold water—the colder the better. Cold water cuts down on the burning pain. Cold water anesthetizes. Cold water encourages the healing process.

The First Commandment—moderation—never leaves us. It is implicit in all of the other commandments—moderate sun, moderate soap and water, moderate cold water. Too much cold water, that is, over-soaking the burned or bruised skin in cold water, is not helping the healing process. Cold, wet compresses are called for.

I have spelled out the need for soaking the skin and for taking warm or cold baths for other skin problems. Soaking may be wrong for burns and bruises, but it may be right for sore and aching feet. A hot footbath with bath salts may be "just what the doctor ordered" for the overworked skin on your feet. The hot water promotes circulation, relieving soreness, while the alkali in the salts help loosen debris, and soften the skin.

Perhaps the most important aspect in "playing it cool" when burns or injuries are involved is your mental coolness. Don't panic. First, anxiety places still another load on the body. Anxiety causes muscles and tissues to tense. Tense muscles and tissues can interfere with natural healing processes.

Second, mental pain inspires the thoughtless impulse to put this or that preparation on the injured area. Chances are that "this and that" will compound the skin problem.

Play it cool: use cold water.

Thou Shalt Not Covet thy Neighbor's VD

The genitals were created for propagation and pleasure. The skin of the vulva and vagina, the skin of the penis, and the skin of the sensual erogenous zones of the body transmit pleasure to the mind via the nerve system.

For the good of that skin, before the mind receives, it should first give.

The mind should give thought to protection from venereal disease: the Sixth Commandment.

The thought of protection from VD should come early in the "game." Should the "game" go that far with that particular person? If it does, what precautions will be taken?

Unfortunately, with the exception of the not-always-effective rubber contraceptive for the man, there are no preventive steps you can take to head off VD, except the also not-always-effective factor of judgment.

Skin problems that arise from human-to-human physical contact are not limited to the sexual organs. Herpes simplex, gonorrhea, and syphilis know no bodily limits.

Post-intercourse vigilance for the male means examining the penis for a drip, being especially alert for a burning sensation when urinating, and checking the body for warts or chancres.

Post-intercourse vigilance for the female can be an exercise in futility. As we previously discussed, signs of VD are not usually discernible to the female carrier of the disease. Only a doctor can know for sure.

The commandment for the female is to go to her physician periodically for checkups, at least annually, but preferably more frequently. Women who are active sexually with different partners should have these professional examinations once a month.

Your Skin Is Not a Private Matter

A fifteen-year-old girl came into my office. She would not tell the nurse the reason for her visit. All she would say was, "It's a skin problem." She seemed embarrassed when I asked her the problem.

"Doctor," she said, pointing to her face, "I have these three blackheads."

A business executive in his forties came in with the same reticence to confide his "mission." When I arrived on the scene, he pointed to a large mole on his right ear.

"That is the side my secretary sits on when I give her dictation, Doctor," he explained. "She keeps looking at the mole. I don't know what she thinks it is, but it is interfering with her accuracy."

Do I scold the teenager for being concerned about three blackheads, or the businessman for being worried about what others think of his mole? Of course not. The pity in both cases is that they were ashamed about their own concern. I never assume an attitude of ridicule toward patients.

My first reaction in such cases is to support the person in the desire to improve the skin. I take care of the matter on the spot, or instruct the patient how to care for the condition. In the case of the teenager, I "scooped" the blackheads out with an extractor and instructed her on how to obtain such a tool and use it herself. In the case of the businessman, I froze the unwanted mole with liquid nitrogen, removed it, and then instructed him on future danger signals he might watch for in other moles on his body.

Do not be embarrassed about wanting to look your best. Vanity is nothing to be ashamed of. It is natural for us to want to look our best. Looking your best also means *being* your best. And health and well-being are matters of survival.

Your skin is your "calling card." The Seventh Commandment is: look your best. Be a skin vigilante, insisting for yourself on a "calling card" that does you justice.

Whether this means a hair transplant, a face lift, or dermabrasion, know what can be done to restore your hair, skin, and nails. Then make the decision. The price you pay for the improvement of your "calling card" may be a lot less than the price you pay otherwise.

Psychiatrists and psychologists know the importance of self-image. How you see yourself can spell the difference between marital, social, and financial success or failure. Do what needs to be done so that you see yourself in the best possible way.

See yourself as capable, successful, dynamic, creative, and attractive.

See to it that your skin permits you to hold that self-image.

Skin Examinations—Amateur and Professional

Esthetic qualities of your skin usually limit self-examination to areas that are your "calling cards"—the face, neck, head, hands, and legs.

Actually, you need to examine all of the skin you live in, but your skin may also merit examination by your physician.

Self-examination is not to be taken lightly. It should be done fastidiously and thoroughly.

Have you ever looked at your anus? If not, you are not alone. Many people have never looked at their anuses. Yet such self-examination with a hand mirror can alert you to problems before they become serious. Warts, skin cancer, and other problems can be seen even when not felt.

An Okinawa bar frequented by United States military men after World War II was run by the glamorous Mama Ginbasha. The restrooms were lined with mirrors—including the toilet bowls!

The upper back is another spot that escapes our casual examination because of difficult access. Even many doctors ignore their patients' backs. They sometimes listen to the chest, but overlook the possibility of skin cancer or other danger signals on the back.

Your first line of defense is yourself. So the Eighth Commandment is: regular self-examination.

The Ninth Commandment is to seek professional advice whenever it seems necessary. Your family doctor is your second line of defense, and behind him are specialists, like the dermatologist and plastic surgeon, as a third line of defense.

Your family doctor can take care of most skin troubles. If he cannot help you, he will know just what specialist can. The plastic surgeon will be recommended for such major projects as dermabrasions, face lifts, buttock lifts, breast shaping, and stomach stretch line or bulge removal. If you have too much skin, he can reduce it or rearrange it. The plastic surgeon can change contours and subcutaneous-based problems like wrinkles. He can get rid of large skin cancers or tumors.

The dermatologist is usually called for all other skin-related matters, such as the skin problems covered in this book.

Now for the most important commandment of all.

Your Psyche and Your Skin

In some countries, especially Japan, the calling card performs a larger function than just serving as a record of name, address, and phone number. The reverse of the card is used to spell out degrees received, honorary positions held, and other information that reflects the stature of the person. Cards are exchanged and read by each party, and the ensuing bows reflect the depth of respect the cards inspire.

As a calling card, the skin is also more than a superficial conveyor of looks. Your skin portrays the state of your inner being.

Your skin is the calling card of your body and soul.

The Tenth Commandment is, in my opinion, the most important of all, because it is the most preventive of skin trouble and the most therapeutic for skin trouble if trouble occurs. Some religionists today refer to the Eleventh Commandment—"Thou Shalt Not Sweat It." That's not bad. It carries the same message as my Tenth Commandment:

Learn how to insulate yourself from emotional shock, and to relax in times of stress.

How does one "learn" this you ask? Good question. And I have what I believe is one answer—biofeedback.

Biofeedback training is a means of getting in control of what has been previously thought to be involuntary or automatic behavior. Biofeedback training is accomplished with the aid of instruments that measure certain physical functions, such as brain waves, muscle tension, and hand or body temperature.

Biofeedback training is being used increasingly to help patients control headaches, hypertension, alcoholism, depression, premenstrual tension, phobias, ulcers, and other symptoms of stress. It has also been found helpful for physical disorders such as cerebral palsy, back trouble, diabetes, and strokes.

Biofeedback training is proving "made to order" for skin problems. By now, you know that most skin disorders, from acne to eczema, are triggered by stress. With biofeedback training, this causative factor is brought under your control, accelerating the benefits of treatment and lessening the chances of recurrence.

Let me give you a picture of what the training is like.

The Potential of Biofeedback for Skin Problems

People have more control over their bodies than they think. In psychosomatic diseases, stress, a mental factor, becomes a physical factor, because the mind runs the body.

True, you say, but this process is automatic. Yes, I say, but thanks to biofeedback, conscious control can be exercised over "automatic" functions.

A doctor takes your temperature, pulse, and blood pressure. He may not even tell you what the results are. In biofeedback, you *are* told what the results are, and you begin to exercise control over your temperature, pulse, and blood pressure.

When Doctor Barbara Brown was conducting her initial research in biofeedback, she worked with a number of persons suffering from a type of colitis. They had no control over their bowels. The colitis was not due to a bug, just to misbehavior of the bowels. These patients always had to be near a bathroom. In these cases, Dr. Brown used a stethoscope as a biofeedback instrument. She let the patients listen to the rumbling of their bowels. They learned very quickly how to control their bowel activity.

Most instruments used today measure skin temperature, muscle tension, and brain waves. The most valuable biofeedback for skin disorders is the brain electroencephalograph. This, connected to your scalp with wires, provides an audio feedback of your brain pulsation rate. As you relax, the beat slows down. The normal active brain wave rate is fourteen to twenty-one pulsations per second. This is called the beta level. As you relax, you enter a peaceful, serene state, a state of tranquility. Here the rate is seven to fourteen pulsations per second.

Whatever you do to relax, you get immediate feedback. By slowing down or speeding up, the machine is teaching you. "Yes, that's right." "No, that's wrong."

You do not have to fall off a bicycle many times to learn how to ride. Biofeedback learning is quicker than learning to ride a bicycle—and far less painful.

Still, biofeedback training is not for everyone. You have to be willing to learn, and then to reinforce. This means a high level of motivation, to make you willing to practice ten minutes a day, twice every day, and to go to weekly sessions—although these procedures vary among practitioners.

Once you master the ability to relax, this ability is useless unless you apply it in your life. Exercise your control when stress strikes.

If you do use biofeedback training, you can not only prevent skin problems, but you can relieve them.

Skin problems react beautifully to biofeedback. In fact, your mirror is a biofeedback instrument teaching you how to mar your complexion with acne and other problems. Irritating life situations—like a flunked exam, a broken date, news of a death—can cause the skin to itch, or the face to break out. Seeing your marred complexion in the mirror causes you even further stress. Now you need to learn how to reverse that procedure.

I have worked on a number of cases with Byron A. Eliashof,

M.D., a psychiatrist who uses biofeedback not only for skin problems, but also for other health problems. We treated patients with such diversified skin problems as herpes simplex of the penis, flat warts, seborrheac dermatitis, and sweat conditions. Every one of our patients responded to some extent to the biofeedback training. Some patients required only three visits, some as many as fifteen. For instance, of the eighteen patients with sweat problems, sixteen responded well and two responded poorly. Desire and cooperation are the keys: there can be no response at all to biofeedback if there is no desire or cooperation from the patient. Unfortunately, this is often the case. Without input from the patient, biofeedback is a useless treatment modality.

How the Skin Responds to Relief from Stress

When a physician shows a sincere interest in the patient's problem, this is also a type of biofeedback. That interest, when backed up with a tolerance for listening and an understanding nature, is excellent therapy.

Neurodermatitis, the skin condition most directly related to "nerves," responds quickly to relaxation. Women get neurodermatitis frequently on the back of the neck—an erogenous zone. In men, neurodermatitis frequently strikes the ankle. Vulvar pruritis is another example of neurodermatitis in women. A woman with vulvar pruritis can't sleep; she scratches away all night. Again, the vulva is an erogenous zone. Apparently, whatever is irritating in life is "salved" by the pleasure of scratching an erogenous zone.

One woman suffering from vulvar pruritis explained that her husband had just died, and she felt sexually frustrated. She did not want to masturbate, so she scratched.

Perianal paritis, an itching anus, is another emotionally disastrous form of neurodermatitis. The bank vice president, sitting at his desk with a client, has to scratch. He has no choice.

Atopic dermatitis, related to asthma, hay fever, and migraine headaches is a general (as opposed to a localized) neurodermatitis. These patients have very strong emotional problems.

Some people are born with "emotional" skin. The skin reacts to their psyche quite sensitively. You can treat emotionally-based skin rashes with cortisone, but the relief will not be permanent unless you treat the psyche.

A nineteen-year-old girl came to see me. She was born with atopic dermatitis. The skin did relatively well until she was fourteen. Then her father died, and the dermatitis flared up. The girl had been suffering with her rashes now for five years. Nothing seemed to work—not creams, ointments, injections, or baths—all of which I prescribed, without results.

Whatever was "feeding" her dermatitis was apparently still in the picture. She had a drug problem, but this was another "effect" of the basic problem, not the cause.

I referred her to a psychiatrist. After a number of sessions, her relationship with her mother emerged as the causative factor of the neurodermatitis. The young woman was advised to move out of the house, and live away from her mother. In two weeks, the improvement on her skin was dramatic. It reflected the "inner" improvement.

In this girl's case, there was a simple solution: move. Compared to this solution, biofeedback would have been a longer, more arduous solution. But it would have worked.

A young man with warts—hundreds of them, multiplying faster than I could keep up with during three years of treatment—was referred by me for biofeedback training, and after fifteen sessions his warts were on the wane.

In this particular case, the skin galvanic response trainer was used. All the patients had to do was learn to relax. The trainer provided a slowed-up sound when the skin reflected this relaxation.

This is the most common biofeedback approach to skin problems. You learn to relax. There is no fooling these machines. You can "let go" physically, but the skin galvanic response will not be dramatic unless you also relax mentally. This is done by countdown techniques, or by imaging techniques involving passive scenes.

Then, the combined mental-physical "posture" of relaxation becomes more automatic the moment such a posture is desired. Practice improves the relaxed response, until finally the patient knows just what to do with the slowing-up sound of the biofeedback equipment. He can relax at will whenever and wherever stress strikes.

When I was at Bellevue Hospital in New York, I had a prisoner-patient who was a psychopathic killer. He had killed people on several occasions. His latest murder, of a little girl in New Jersey, had been committed just before I was called in to treat him for lichen planus. Lichen planus is a rare skin disease where the sufferer gets raised reddish-purple patches just about anywhere on the body. The murderer had patches on his lips, mouth, wrist, penis, anus, and a few other places. They itched "murderously."

Every time he was interviewed, interrogated, or brought before a judge, the prisoner's lichen planus flared up. His stress was beyond biofeedback training, or any other approach. All I could do was to give him massive doses of cortisone, to keep him comfortable enough to respond to questioning at hearings. This man was later committed to a mental institution. I do not know the outcome—but I'll wager that his lichen planus provided a convenient "barometer" for measuring the effectiveness of psychiatric treatment in normalizing his emotional "climate."

Relax, and your skin responds.

If your skin is healthy skin, it will become even healthier.

On the other hand, if your guilt and self-punishment are being expressed through neurotic excoriation—that is, itching and scratching. . . .

Or, if your pent up feelings of hostility and aggression are being expressed through trichotillomania and scratching. . . .

Or, if your masochistic tendencies are being expressed through disfigurement and excessive scratching. . . .

In the above cases, your skin will respond to relief from the stresses by alleviating the conditions that cause itching and scratching.

Your Skin's Impressive IQ

I have always been intrigued by the skin. Of course, that is why I became a dermatologist. But now, with every passing decade I grow more and more in awe of this marvelous living organ of the human body.

Your heart, your liver, your kidneys, your lungs—these, too, are organs with tremendous abilities. And what about your brain! But somehow, the skin you live in continues to impress me more and more, as I watch it respond to the inner and outer environment.

The skin is your outer periphery. Yet the skin seems closest to you. Your psyche and skin are in intimate touch. The skin your body lives in is the skin your psyche lives in, too; but perhaps your psyche is a more than equal tenant.

Love, and your skin warms.

Tense, and your skin sweats.

Fear, and the hair follicles rise.

Be embarrassed, and the blood vessels dilate.

Our skin shakes and shivers when necessary to keep us warm.

Our skin eliminates or absorbs—"knowing" what to do.

Our skin is a veritable chemical laboratory that comes up with exactly the right things to keep us well and functioning properly.

If you could give the organs of the body an intelligence test, of course the brain would place first. But the skin would probably place a close second.

Respect your skin as I do. Some of us are our skins' worst enemy.

Perhaps it is fitting for me to end this "house call" by reminding you how to be your skin's best friend:

- Treat your skin in moderation.
- Protect your skin from excessive exposure to strong sunlight.
- Use soap and water to keep your skin clean.
- Know your lotions and cosmetics.
- Play it "cool" in treating your skin for burn or injury.
- Be aware of and avoid exposure to venereal disease.
- Help your skin to look its best.
- Examine your total skin periodically.

- Seek professional care for your skin when indicated.

And—for the sake of your psyche and your skin:

- Counteract life's stresses with superior serenity.

Index

About the Author

Dr. Norman Goldstein has been practicing dermatology for fifteen years, and he is a fellow of both the American Academy of Dermatology and the American College of Physicians.

An associate professor at the Medical School of the University of Hawaii, Dr. Goldstein has lectured at universities in New York, California, Chicago, and Miami. He received his M.D. from the State University of New York, and also attended New York University and Columbia University.

Dr. Goldstein has published articles in numerous medical journals, including the *Journal of the American Medical Association and the Archives of Dermatology*.